PRINCETON SERIES ON THE MIDDLE EAST

Bernard Lewis and Andrá[illegible]mori, Editors

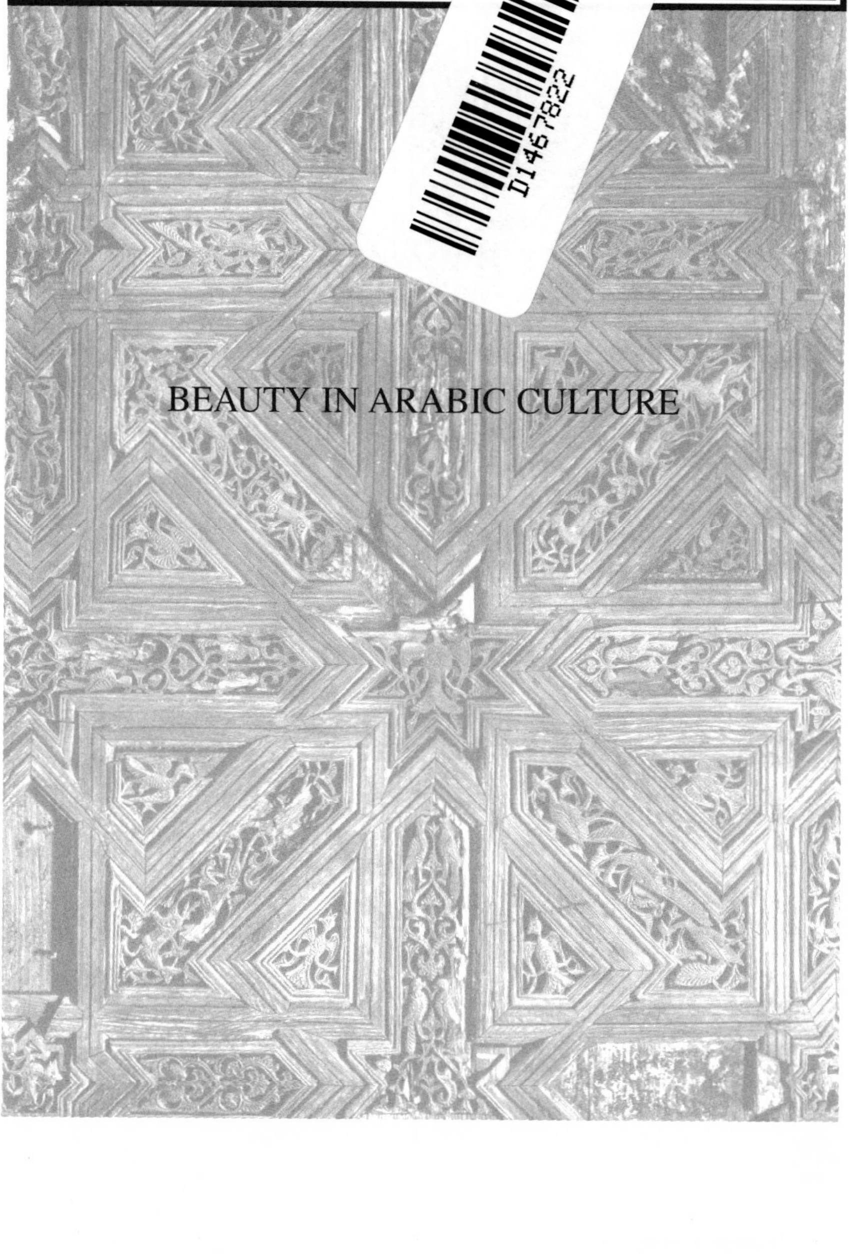

BEAUTY IN ARABIC CULTURE

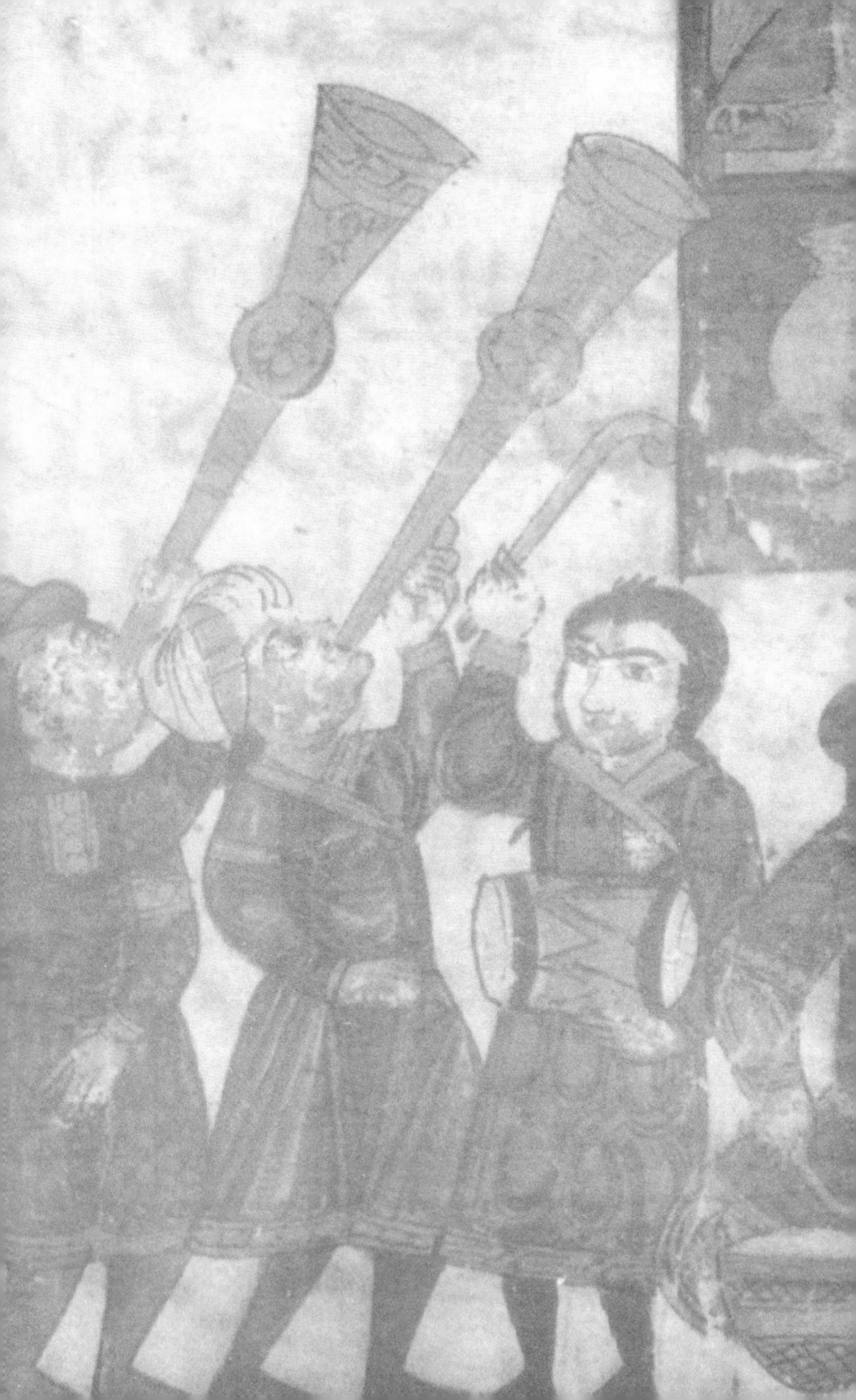

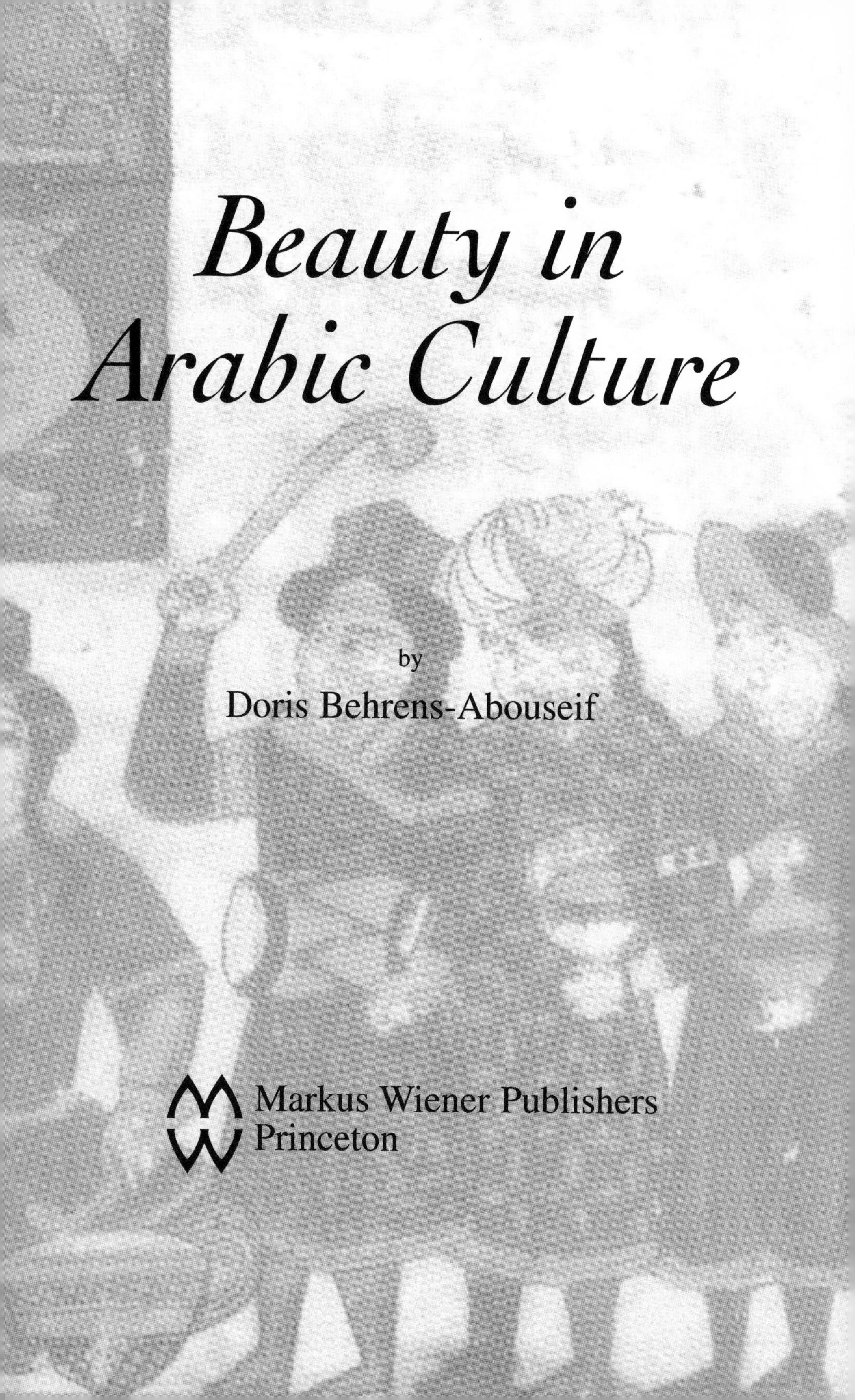

Beauty in Arabic Culture

by

Doris Behrens-Abouseif

Markus Wiener Publishers
Princeton

Cover photo: Dome of the Rock (Courtesy Aramco World)

Frontispiece: Cappella Palatina, Museo Nazionale, Palermo
(Courtesy Oleg Grabar)

First American edition, 1999

For information write to: Markus Wiener Publishers
231 Nassau Street, Princeton, NJ 08542

Book Design: Cheryl Mirkin
Photo Consultant: Cynthia Robinson

Library of Congress Cataloging-in-Publication Data

Behrens-Abouseif, Doris.
[Schönheit in der arabischen Kultur. English]
Beauty in Arabic culture by Doris Behrens-Abouseif.
(Princeton series on the Middle East)
Includes bibliographical references and index.
ISBN 1-55876-198-5 hardcover
ISBN 1-55876-199-3 paper
1. Aesthetics, Arab. 2. Civilization, Arab. 3. Civilization, Islamic.
I. Title. II. Series.
BH221 1998
111'.85'09174927—dc21 98-43118 CIP

Markus Wiener Publishers books are printed in the United States of America on acid-free paper, and meet the guidelines for permanence and durability of the Committee on Production Guidelines for Book Longevity of the Council on Library Resources.

For Gerhard Behrens

Inna likulli shay'in ḥilya.

(*Everything has its ornament*)

Ḥadīth

The art that is frankly decorative is the art to live with.

Oscar Wilde

Contents

Introduction

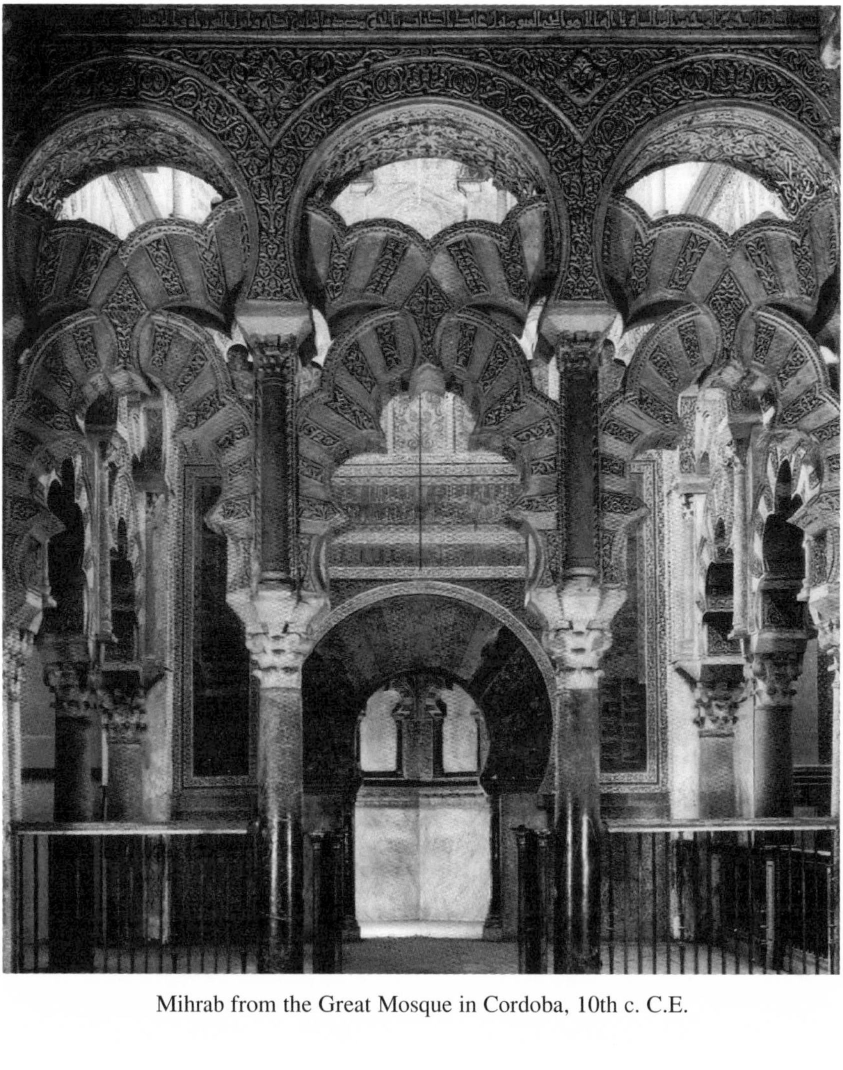

Mihrab from the Great Mosque in Cordoba, 10th c. C.E.

The *Encyclopaedia of Islam* includes an entry under the heading "*ʿilm al-d̲jamāl*"[1] (the modern Arabic equivalent of aesthetics), in which we read that a general theory on aesthetics and "precise definitions for the terms used in this field are lacking in the history of Arabic civilization." This lack of aesthetic conceptualization is not exclusive to Islamic culture; it is also characteristic of other pre-modern cultures. Umberto Eco, among other historians of aesthetics, notes that the European Middle Ages also never developed a theory of fine arts to deal with artistic creations whose essential purpose was to convey aesthetic enjoyment, with all the exalted meanings involved in such an aspiration.

There is a discrepancy between the practical attitude of the Muslims toward the arts, which allowed aesthetics to be a norm of life, and the absence of a general theory of the arts in their culture. The visual arts were enjoyed and promoted almost everywhere and at all times in the Muslim world. Architecture has always been one of the most prominent forms of Islamic art, but as has been repeated many times, Islamic culture produced no theoretical writings equivalent to those of Vitruvius in classical Europe or to the Indian *vastushastras* that controlled or analyzed the process of architectural design and execution. What De Bruyne writes in his eminent study of medieval European aesthetics, "The fact that the medieval authors did not develop a systematic theory of the arts does not mean that they were not aware of the relationship between art and beauty,"[2] is also valid for the Muslim world.

Whereas an important body of literature, based on the analysis of philosophical and theological texts, has been written on classical and medieval European concepts of beauty, little has been done in the same field for Arab-Islamic studies, if we except works devoted to Islamic art that also include a discussion of aesthetic matters. Historians of literature have dealt extensively with aesthetic concepts in the specific context of Arabic classical literature, but this subject has yet to be tackled from the philosophical or social point of view, as it has been in medieval European studies.

The art-historical approach to aesthetics tends to be global. Taking as its point of departure the Islamic phenomenon of design, it seeks to encompass the whole of the Muslim world from Central Asia to Spain in an evolution from the 8th to the 18th century or later, a perspective too broad and too general to be adopted in an investigation based on literary sources. Therefore, this study will use not an art-historical approach, but rather a cultural perspective that relies largely on Arabic literary sources. It is thus necessary to restrict the scope of this study to Arabic culture instead of encompassing the entire Muslim world.

Classical Islam was Arabic-speaking and Arabic-writing. The great translation activity of Greek philosophy and science and their elaboration in the Arabic language made Arabic the language of Islamic philosophy. The first steps of Islamic culture took place under Arab hegemony and patronage. Its golden age was the time when Baghdad was the capital of the Abbasid caliphate and the center of the Muslim world, and Arabic was the language of its intellectual discourse. The political centrifugal movements of the 9th century did not weaken the cultural creativity of the Abbasid melting pot; on the contrary, the Abbasid golden age has been called by A. Mez the Renaissance of Islam. The term is problematic taken in its literal meaning of a revival of something that had waned, because the golden age represented the birth of a new culture, not the rebirth of an old one. But the term renaissance is appropriate if we define it as the birth of a culture comparable to that of the European Renaissance which, with its enlightened and inquisitive mind, generated an outburst of creativity in the arts and sciences. The Abbasid period brought forth most of the criteria that shaped and defined Arab-Islamic culture, theology, literature, the rational sciences, philosophy, musicology, and even ways of life for centuries to come. The major features of Islamic art—calligraphy, geometry, the arabesque, and *muqarnas*—were established in this period. The artistic norms set then have prevailed throughout the entire pre-modern history of the Muslim world.

Another good reason for limiting this investigation to Arabic culture is that Arabic belles-lettres and literary criticism played an important role in the formulation of aesthetic criteria. Poetry has always been the art most cherished and most extensively discussed by the Arabs, who produced a tremendous literature in literary criticism. Sufism, which played an important role in all Muslim societies of the post-classical age, including literature, took diverse forms following regional, political, and cultural particularities. In Arabic literature sufism did not play the paramount role it did in Iran, nor did Arabic sufi poetry attain the importance and quality it did in the Persian language. The greatest Arab poets, al-Mutanabbī (d. 965) and Abū 'l-ʿAlāʾ al-Maʿarrī (d. 1058), were pessimistic intellectuals. They were neither religious nor mystics. On the other hand, the Iranian *Book of Kings* (Firdawsī's [d. 1020] *Shāhnāme*) and Niẓāmī's [d. 1141] poetical work), which had a strong impact on Iranian and Turkish literature and art, had no influence on the Arabic artistic tradition. Ibn Khaldūn's (d. 1406) rationalistic vision of history was an outgrowth of the tremendous historiographical movement that Arab culture of the late medieval period produced.

Sufi thought followed altogether different regional trends. Suhrawardī (d. 1191) and his metaphysics of light had a stronger influence on the Iranian than on the Arab world, which adopted a more sober form of sufism, under the influence of the enlightened orthodox theology of al-Ghazālī (d. 1111). Ibn ʿArabī (d. 1240), with his esoteric mysticism, had a more pronounced influence on Turkish, Iranian, and Indian than on Arab sufism. The Persian poet Jalāl al-Dīn Rūmī (d. 1273), often identified as most representative of Islamic mysticism, had little impact on Arabic culture.

The Mongol invasion changed the configuration of the Muslim world and increased the dissimilarities between its eastern and western parts. The subsequent period produced a more conservative culture in the Arabic-speaking world. Its learning and scholarship became institutionalized, producing pragmatic rather than speculative sciences, such as encyclopaedic and historical literature. Various disciplines lost their appeal; philosophy was rejected, and a moderate sufism was promoted instead. The classical Abbasid heritage, however, was never repudiated by late medieval Arab society. Rather, it was perpetuated through the tremendous book production of the following centuries, which brought forth, with untiring zeal, copies of old texts that were also integrated into new anthologies and encyclopaedic literature. This conservative attitude safeguarded norms and ideals once set, even though they had been superseded by new, more puritanic trends. If the Mamluk period did not produce new dictionaries on musicians or physicians, for instance, the earlier ones continued to be used; they were consulted, copied, quoted, and discussed well into the Ottoman period.

Islamic Iranian and Turkish culture began to flourish as Arab hegemony was declining; they evolved in a different direction, driven by historical factors different from those that affected the Arabic-speaking world. The artistic experience manifested in the arts of the Ottomans, Timurids, Safavids and Moghuls had no parallel in the Maghreb or Egypt and Syria, which remained largely faithful to their medieval traditions. Painting, and the figural representations it involves, disappeared almost entirely in the arts of the Arab region after the 14th century. A discussion of artistic concepts cannot, therefore, be indiscriminately applied to the entire Muslim world. By the time the Iranians had revived their own literary language and culture, their cultural influence on the Arabic-speaking peoples, which attained its apogee in the Abbasid period, had diminished. When the Ottomans conquered the Arab lands in the 16th century, their cultural influence was minimal, and Arabic continued to be the official and literary language.

As Ibn Khaldūn admitted, Arabic culture was largely shaped by non-Arabs. The criterion for defining Arabic culture here is thus linguistic and not ethnic. Arabic, as the language of the Koran, i.e., of God, continues to be a cultural link across the Muslim world. The term Arabic culture in this book therefore always means the Arabic-speaking world, to which belong not only the present Arab nations but also Muslim Spain and the Arabic-writing Iran of the classical age. This terminology is comparable to using the term "Iranian art and culture" to refer to a culture to which Turkic peoples also belong. The role of the Arabic language was similar to that of Latin in medieval Europe, with the important difference that, unlike Latin, Arabic remains a living language. On many occasions, however, whenever a distinction between Arabic and Islamic cannot be made, the term "Islamic" will be used. Otherwise when speaking of Arabic culture we are referring to an Arabic-speaking cosmopolitan culture to which indigenous Christians and Jews also contributed.

In the absence of a general theory of aesthetics, the meaning of art or beauty in Muslim society has to be deduced from scattered literary and cultural statements in addition to the works of art themselves. The written statements relevant to this study are found in a wide variety of sources, including the Koran, legal, religious, and sufi texts, chronicles, biographies, belles-lettres, literary criticism, and scientific, geographical, and philosophical literature. The *Arabian Nights*, which were collected and written down in the late medieval Arab world, mainly in Egypt, are, despite their disparate origins, a significant document for the understanding of Arabic aesthetics.

The statements about beauty presented in this book therefore encompass religious, intellectual, and literary ideals, reveal artistic sensibilities and norms of life, and elucidate the social context of artistic production.

This book follows not a chronological structure, but a typological one, in a panoramic view of constant and characteristic themes, referring only in individual cases to historical developments or mutations. Consequently, it is not concerned with the analysis of origins and roots of concepts or artistic forms that have been adopted by and integrated into Arabic culture. When dealing with a subject as broad as concepts of beauty in a culture over centuries, compression and generalization are obligatory. In order to make observations or statements defining how beauty was conceived, or what art meant to a medieval society, it is necessary to concentrate on the cultural mainstream, leaving out exceptions to the rules.

Studies of European medieval concepts of beauty have inspired many of the questions raised in this book. The questions raised by Oleg Grabar in recent years on the subject of beauty and pleasure in Islamic art, as well as conversations with him, have also stimulated my work. Western scholars' statements on the meaning of Islamic art, which have been consulted and used for this study, will not be discussed; they deserve a separate study dealing with the sociology of Orientalism. Neither is it my aim to analyze Arabic concepts of beauty based on modern aesthetic criteria, but merely to compile and present pre-modern Arabic statements related to the subject of beauty.

Medieval European and Islamic philosophical thought have many similarities and common traditions. However, a major difference that struck me has prompted the writing of this book: the separation between the good and the beautiful in Arabic culture, and the appreciation of beauty in poetry and the visual arts for its own sake, without commitment to religious or moral criteria, an attitude uncommon in medieval Europe but one that anticipates modernity.

The Religious Approach

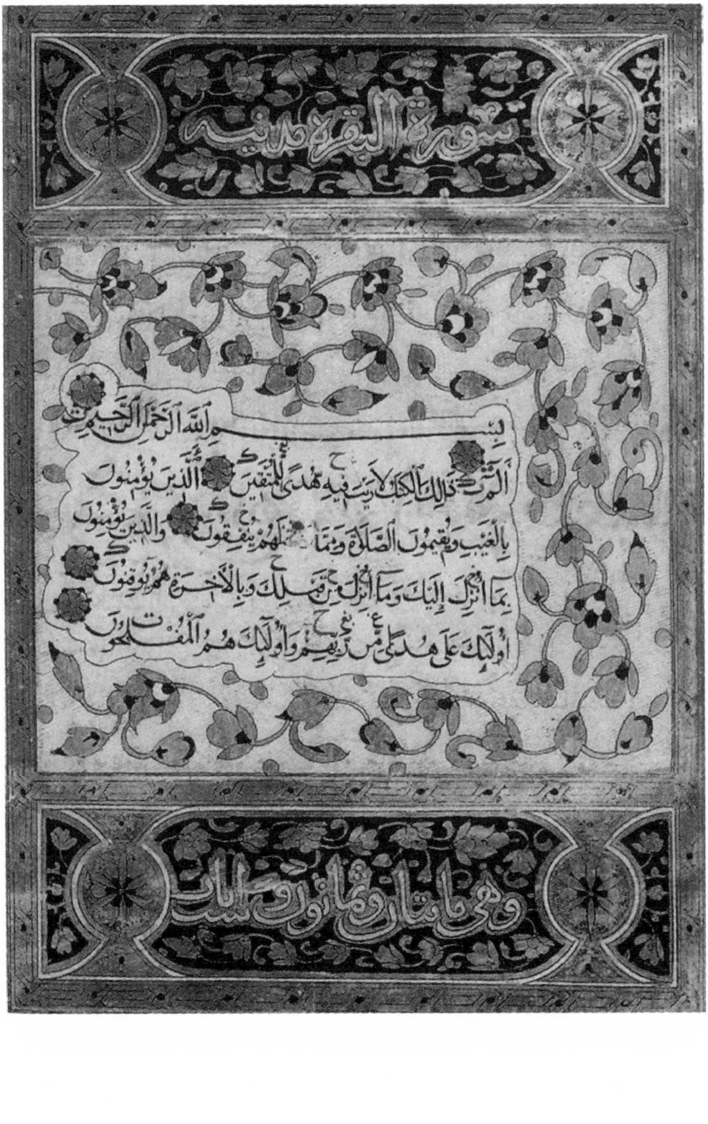

The Image of the World

A study of Arabic-Islamic concepts of beauty is bound to turn up parallels with medieval European thought, as Islamic and the European cultures have common roots in both biblical tradition and Hellenic civilization, and because medieval European thought was directly and substantially influenced by Islamic philosophy. The Arabs, however, did not adopt the whole Greek package. They left out many subjects that were alien to their culture or did not appeal to them (such as Homer and the theater), and they were not influenced by Latin literature; Vitruvius and Seneca are not to be found in Arabic sources. Despite their veneration of Aristotle, the Muslims did not look back nostalgically on Greek culture like the West, but sought merely to learn from it and add it to their own knowledge.

Philosophy fulfilled a different function in the West than it did in Islam. In Europe it encompassed ordinary religious life and served the church, while in the Arab world it remained a matter for elite intellectuals. Muslim philosophers considered philosophy a subject exclusively for intellectuals and not part of common religious practice. Attempts to reconcile Greek philosophy with Islam were ultimately unsuccessful, and philosophers such as Ibn Sīnā and Ibn Rushd regarded the domains of philosophy and religion as separate. Eventually, Arabic religious thought even refuted Greek philosophy as incompatible with Islam, and turned to sufism instead as the alternative to the legalistic approach of Muslim orthodoxy. Sufism, although it includes Platonic and Neoplatonic as well as Oriental elements, could be more easily integrated into Muslim religious practice because of the non-programmatic and individual nature of its approach and because, unlike philosophy, it had an important populist component in which philosophical thought was diluted.

The main contributions of the Greek philosophical heritage to Muslim Arabic culture were the Aristo-platonic and Neoplatonic doctrines of emanation, which conceived an eternal world ruled by the eternal One. All things emanated from him and gravitated around him, attracted by love or desire. The soul, by freeing itself from the body and by ascending toward absolute beauty and truth, could return to the One with the help of the Active Intelligence that serves as an intermediary between the spiritual and the material world. This doctrine, however, collided with orthodox Islam when it reached the Koranic concept of creation *ex nihilo* and the Muslim belief in the resurrection of the body. Islamic theology agreed with philosophy, however, on the relation in human existence between soul and matter and on the concept that the immaterial and immortal soul is the principle of life and movement. With intelligence, which is a faculty of the soul, human beings aspire to perfection and to God. They must free their souls and fight against the material powers of the lower universe. The fact that orthodox Islam detached itself from philosophy did not prevent philosophy from exerting a tremendous influence on Islam. Even the most categorical antagonist of the philosophical approach, Ghazālī, did not escape the influence of Aristotle and Ibn Sīnā, using their methods to generate his own concepts.

Islam is religion and state, or religion and life (*dīn wa dawla, dīn wa dunyā*), which means that it comprehends both the spiritual and the social aspects of human life. The Koran includes not only religious truth but the regulation of worship and of human and social behavior. Islam is a religion of law, and its theology is essentially based on jurisprudence. The *Sharīʿa* transmits the will of God and rules every aspect of human life; it sets down precepts of the faith which the Muslim has a duty to follow. It was natural under these circumstances that Muslim society eventually turned to sufism as an outlet. With its ecstatic and intimate approach to God and its search for the immediate religious experience, sufism offered an alternative to the ritual and legalistic character of the *Sharīʿa*.

Human beings are created in God's image to serve and represent Him on earth; they must submit to God's power, which is absolute and beyond comprehension. According to the prevailing doctrine of al-Ashʿarī (d. 935), God's creation is constant and permanent; He is the creator and the cause of all things, good and evil; He also created the acts of human beings but gave them in addition the capacity to acquire the responsibility for their deeds. The acquired power to act (*kasb*) was a compromise that had to be formulated as a response to the principle of free will advocated by the rationalistic Muʿtazilites in the 9th century, and which consensus ultimately refuted.

Asharʿist doctrine holds that the Muslim has to believe the Koran without question. The Koran is uncreated and, as an eternal attribute of God, it is immutable. Even though some anthropomorphic attributes of God formulated in the Koran—such as His sitting on a throne and having hands and a face, seeing and hearing—may be difficult for a believer to grasp, they have to be taken on faith, without asking how (*bilā kayfa*). They should not be interpreted allegorically, as advocated by the rationalist school of the Muʿtazilites.

Sunni thought refutes the allegorical interpretation of the Koran favored by the philosophers and the rationalists. The language of the Koran is direct and concrete; it does not use metaphysical terms. Paradise, for example, as described in the Koran with all its worldly features, is taken literally and not symbolically by the majority of orthodox theologians. The Koran prophesies physical resurrection, not mere immortality. Consensus had it that Paradise would be a place of carnal delights as described in the holy text. In his critique of the philosophical approach, Ghazālī wrote that it was imperative

> to refute their denial of the resurrection of the body and the return of the soul to its physical frame, the existence of a physical hell, the existence of paradise and the houris, and the rest of what mankind has been promised, together with their assertion that all that is mere parable is coined for the common people and intended to connote a spiritual reward and retribution, these being higher in rank than the corporeal. This is contrary to the beliefs of all Muslims.[3]

Unlike the philosophers, who preferred to interpret Koranic descriptions of paradise as a parable, orthodox scholars believed in the compatibility of spiritual and bodily happiness. On the whole, Islam has always advocated moderation and rejected excess, addressing the believer as a member of society rather than as a solitary worshiper. For the orthodox Muslim, supreme happiness can be reached only in paradise after it has been earned in this world; for the philosopher and the mystic, excellence and happiness were to be pursued in this life by exalting the soul and its intelligence.

The word of God, the Koran, is a book open to everyone; it has to be interpreted word for word; its exegesis is guided by a juridical and semantic mind. Because the orthodox interpretation of the Koran leaves little room for allegory, Sunni Muslim culture did not develop a symbolic repertoire, neither did it need a clergy to solve mysteries or interpret allegories.

The Prophet Muḥammad was a human being, with all human attributes, whom God selected to be His messenger on earth. Although Muslim tradition views the Prophet as an outstanding personality, and sufis venerate him as a symbol of revelation, he is not believed to have been involved in the wording of the Koran or to have had supernatural attributes. Muḥammad was illiterate. As Massignon said, the Koran is to Muslims what Jesus, and not the Bible, is to Christians. God manifests Himself in His book and in His creation. The universe, with its beauty and perfection, is full of signs that reveal the Creator. These signs are directly legible and perceivable by the faithful; they need no religious authority's mediation. To recognize God's signs is a matter of cognition (*maʿrifa, ʿilm). Maʿrifa* is often used by the sufis to mean the perception of God; *ʿilm* is more complex and includes the profane sciences as well. Knowledge in Islam is equivalent to faith in Christianity; according to the sufis, with real knowledge (*maʿrifa*) man can move mountains.[4] It is the highest virtue and the highest duty man can pursue, and it is the way to individual happiness.[5] God is the most Knowledgeable. The fact that God's word reaches humanity through a book rather than through a person helped to give Islamic culture its intellectual character; reading and learning are essential to religion.

The Islamic community was intellectually more heterogeneous in its earlier than in its later history. In the 9th century the rationalistic Muʿtazilites initiated a debate concerning the problem of human free will versus God's determination that ended up with the triumph of Ashʿarī's compromise. Sunni Islam, because of its social orientation, has always tended toward compromise and the reconciliation of opposing ideas. Ashʿarī and Ghazālī were the two thinkers with the most decisive impact on Arabic Sunni thought, and the merit of both was to achieve a synthesis reconciling major opposing principles that could have seriously split the community. Ashʿarī mitigated the conflict between the fatalistic and the extremists among the rationalistic schools by presenting a doctrine of

Koranic interpretation that did not rely on *ratio* alone, but also left room for faith. Ghazālī's role was to reconcile orthodoxy with sufism and end speculative philosophical thought.

After the 10th century and once Sunnism had acquired its essential features, jurists and theologians agreed that individual theological endeavors (*ijtihād*) should continue no longer and that they should rather concentrate their efforts on applying the laws already elaborated: the door to individual reasoning was closed. This should not be understood as a categorical prohibition, but as a principle that over time became more strongly applied.

In spite of the supreme role of the *Sharīʿa,* Muslim society did acknowledge the existence of domains that could be ruled by regulations other than religious laws, so long as they did not conflict with Islam. For instance, the rational sciences inherited from the Greeks continued to be acknowledged even after philosophy was rejected by orthodox authorities. *Siyāsa* (statecraft) was also acknowledged as a source of legislation to be adopted by the monarch for leading the community. *Siyāsa* is distinct from religious law, but complementary to it, and should not conflict with it.[6]

In Islam, adherence to the community of believers and the requirements of the collective are preponderant; personal ideas are subordinated to the collective and its tradition. The Prophet's sayings and acts, codified as *Ḥadīth*, had the authority to serve as precedents and guidelines for the conduct of individuals and the community. The *Ḥadīth* is included in the *sunna* (tradition), which is a fundamental legal source, second in importance only to the Koran. The preservation and transmission of the Prophet's traditions and the early history of the Muslim community were matters of major concern to the religious authorities. Islamic ideals aspired to the restoration of original Islam as it was at the time when the Prophet and his companions governed the life of the first community. As a result, Muslim society has always been guided by the obligation to know and study its past. The study of history, which can be supported by several passages in the Koran inciting the believer to look into the past for models of behavior, is a moral duty. As a result the amount of Arabic historiographical literature is immense.

The focus on the past and on the origins of Islam, along with the closing of the door to individual reasoning, contributed to the static character of Arabic pre-modern culture. Nostalgia determined many aspects of culture. Von Grunebaum uses the term "chronological primitivism" to characterize the Arab image of the world,[7] which looks back to the golden age and finds decline or moral decay in the present. The best Arabic poetry is pessimistic. The Arabic language, the pride of the Arabs, is believed to be represented in its unsurpassable beauty in the Koran, and therefore it was, and still is, the model for literary excellence. Even on the profane level of poetry, the criteria of excellence were believed to have been attained and set in the pre-Islamic poetic tradition. This nostalgic approach led to a lack of flexibility, and even to hostility toward radical innovation and free thinking.

In spite of this nostalgic bent, Arabic culture was not exclusively oriented toward the past. By urging people to contemplate the universe in order to recognize the signs of divine creation, the Koran stimulated great interest in knowledge and epistemology within Islamic culture. Knowledge is essential for the perception of God and thus an aspect of religion.

The Koran and the Universe

"God is beautiful and loves all beauty" is a saying attributed to the Prophet that is quoted as often today as it was in medieval times. Scholars of Islamic theology and exegetes may doubt the authenticity of this *ḥadīth,* many discarding it as apocryphal, but this does not shake its validity and importance for Islamic culture. That the concept of God's beauty is Platonic and not Semitic also does not invalidate its significance.[8] This *ḥadīth* has been of basic importance to sufi thought, and it is an integral part of both intellectual and popular Islamic belief.

The term for beauty (*ḥusn* or *jamāl*) is not frequently used in the Koran; *jamīl* (beautiful) is used but in a moral context, referring to fortitude (*ṣabr*). It has been said that Arabic, like many languages, does not discriminate between beautiful and good.[9] The verb *zayyana,* however, which is used in the Koran, means to make beautiful, to embellish, or to ornament, and therefore it refers essentially to aesthetic beauty. Another term for beautiful is *malīḥ*, deriving from the root *m-l-ḥ*, which forms the word *milḥ* meaning salt. It implies the notion of the beautiful as having salt added to it, or being spicy, which is closer to delectability than to moral good. The word *wasīm* refers only to human physical beauty. The Koran is full of references to the visual beauty of the world, inviting the believer to contemplate the universe in order to recognize the signs of God's majesty.

The Koran itself, through the uniqueness of its language, is such a sign. The Muslims praise the beauty of the Koran as God's own words. Its uniqueness is evidenced by its inimitability; no human is capable of composing anything equivalent or comparable to it.[10] The evidence for the divinity of the Koran is its beauty. As Kirmani wrote, we are dealing here with an "ästhetischer Gottesbeweis," i.e., beauty as proof of the Koran's divine source.[11] The basic Muslim belief that the Koran is unique refers not only to its content, but to its form as well, ascribing an aesthetic value to the word of God in a concept unparalleled in other religions. The Koran is not only revelation, but literature and art as well. Its beauty is mani-

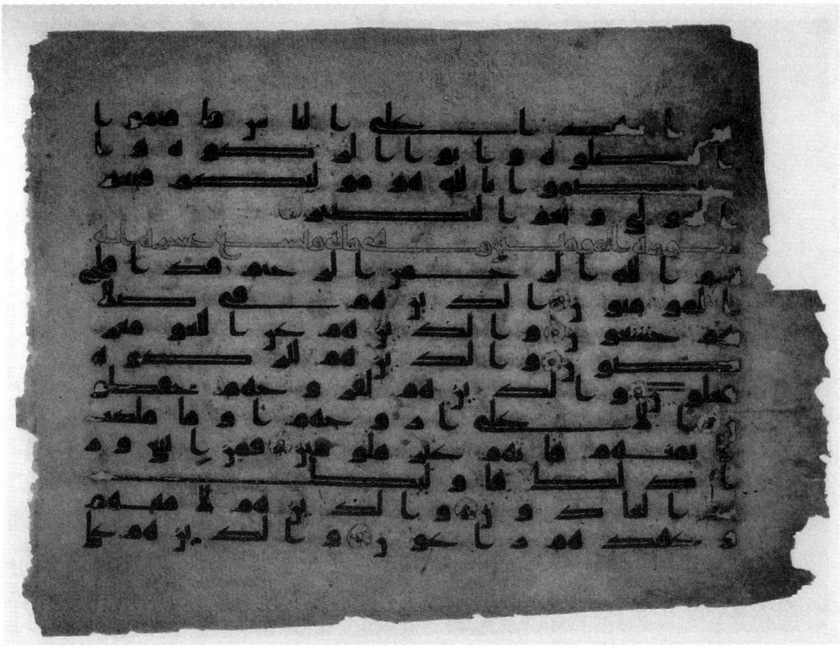

Kufic Koran, Syria, 9th century. Bayerische Staatsbibliothek, Munich.

fested by its enjoyable character. A *ḥadīth* says: *laysa minnā man lam yataghanna bi'l-qur'ān* ("nobody can escape the pleasure of the Koran")[12] (the word *yataghannā* originally means to enjoy music). Facing opposition from the puritanical side, however, theologians have argued that the Koran is both a revelation and a source of enjoyment and that there is no contradiction between the two. The fact that orthodox theologians do not acknowledge translations of the Koran as authentic texts attests to the importance attached to its form and to the power of its textual beauty, especially when it is recited.

According to Ghazālī, some passages in the Koran can induce ecstasy (*wajd*) in the listener; for this reason the performance of religious music should be authorized as a form of worship. Muslim tradition described the ecstasy conveyed by the Koran to the listener, in terms similar to those referring to the enjoyment of poetry; listeners would weep or lose consciousness just upon hearing the Koran recited. Many accounts from the early Islamic period tell about persons who were converted to Islam after hearing Koran recitation, so enchanted were they by the beauty of its sound.

Unlike the Christians who pursue redemption from original sin, Muslims have a positive attitude to worldly life; they see death not as punishment but as part of the divine order to which man submits. "Prayer was supplication and not expiation," comments M. Dols on Muslim reaction to the Black Death.[13] The Prophet himself was the model for a virtuous man who enjoyed life. Muslim ethics tended less toward the Platonic rejection of the body than toward the Aristotelian conciliatory view that the fate of the human soul is linked to that of the body. The search for happiness is conditioned by people's worldly needs.[14] In Sunni Islam there is no room for martyrdom, in the Christian sense of achieving salvation through suffering for the faith.[15] Muslims can enjoy God's creation and worship Him without having to be in conflict with their own nature. God's creation is intrinsically good and beautiful and invites humanity to enjoy it within certain ethical rules. The terminology used in the Koran to convey the beauty of the universe, far from being metaphysical, is rather concrete and direct.[16]

> Did you not see how God sent down water from the sky with which we brought forth fruits of different hues? In the mountains there are streams of various shades of red and white, and jet-black rocks. Men, beasts, and cattle have their different colors too. (35:27, 28)

> He is the Mighty One, the Merciful, who excelled in the creation of all things. (32:7)

> . . . God, who has perfected all things. (27:88)

> Turn up your eyes: can you detect a single crack? Then look once more and yet again: your eyes will in the end grow dim and weary. (67:3, 4)

> We have decked the heavens with constellations and made them lovely to behold. (15:17, 18)

The word *zayyana* (to adorn) is often used in the Koran in the context of God adorning the universe with His creation:

> We have decked the earth with all manner of ornaments. . . (18:7)[17]

> Have they never observed the sky above them, and marked how We built it up and furnished it with ornaments, leaving no crack in its expanse? (50:6)

> We have adorned the lowest heaven with lamps. . . (67:5)

Not only was nature created to please, but human beings are entitled to ornament themselves to be agreeable. When God created the universe he provided humanity with material to exploit for jewelry and adornment:

> We have given you clothes to cover your nakedness, and garments pleasing to the eye. . . (7:25)

> It is He who has subjected to you the ocean, so that you may eat of its fresh fish and bring from its depth ornaments with which you adorn your persons. (16:14)

> From both (seas) you eat fresh fish and bring up ornaments to deck yourselves with. (35:12)

Life in Paradise also involves luxury and ornamentation:

> . . . they shall be decked with bracelets of gold, and arrayed in garments of fine green silk and rich brocade. (18:30)

> You shall be served with golden dishes and golden cups. (43:71)

> They shall be arrayed in garments of fine green silk and rich brocade, and adorned with bracelets of silver. (76:21)

These Koranic verses praise the beauty of the universe, showing that it was created to be enjoyed and that ornament was an integral attribute of beauty. Ornament as an expression of refinement is a part of natural and human beauty. Jewelry and decoration are not superfluous artificial additions, they are part of God's creation. Theologians often speak of *tazyīn al-arḍ*, which means "the adornment of the earth," by God, and they describe virtues as an "adornment" of humanity. If western Christians described God as the architect of the universe, the Muslims implicitly present Him as an artist who made the universe beautiful and pleasing and spoke the Koran in a most poetic and fascinating language.

On the other hand, the Koran also uses the word *zīna* (adornment) to represent vanity, describing this world as a game, or pastime, and adornment, all of which are illusions. Adornment in this case epitomizes the worthlessness of ephemerality, a view dear to sufis:

> Know that the life of this world is but a sport and a pastime, a show and an empty vaunt (*zīna*) among you, a quest for riches and more children. It is like the plants that flourish after rain: the husbandman rejoices to see them grow, but then they wither and run yellow, soon becoming worthless stubble. (57:20)

Ghazālī, the Sufi Way, and the Symbolism of Light

AL-GHAZĀLĪ

Abū Ḥāmid al-Ghazālī (d. 1111),[18] jurist, theologian, and mystic, is a towering figure in Sunni Islam. He vehemently defended orthodoxy against Shīʿa doctrines and Neoplatonic philosophy, and advocated the sufi experience as the highest form of knowledge. His philosophy deals with spiritual as well as with temporal beauty. His discourse on this subject is nuanced sometimes to the point of ambivalence. Quoting statements by the Prophet, he condemned the decoration of mosques because it diverted the worshiper's attention, and because, according to a tradition, the angel Gabriel ordered Muḥammad to build a mosque in Medina without decoration.[19] Ghazālī also condemned the illumination of Koranic fascicles. Speaking of human beauty, he warned against the seduction that can lead to sin.[20] At the same time, however, unlike other orthodox theologians, he did not condemn music altogether, but encouraged its religious performance. All beauty that can be perceived in this world by sight, ear, or mind is, according to him, a reflection of God's light and His power. All that is beautiful, lovable, and good is a manifestation of His majesty. God combines all the attributes of beauty and perfection and therefore He deserves all our love.

Ghazālī draws a parallel between human beings' perception of God's creation and their perception of art. Just as a beautiful calligraphy or a wall painting inspires the beholder to reflect upon the artist's talent, so the wonders of the world induce us to think of Him who designed it. In long passages Ghazālī invites the believer to contemplate the beauty of the universe, of the human body, of nature and its fauna, comparing the world with a big house decorated with the most precious materials. A very significant feature of Ghazālī's statement on beauty is that he does not qualify the universe as beautiful *a priori* because it is God's creation, but rather expects human beings to perceive this beauty through contemplation and reflection, which will lead them ultimately to God. The perception of beauty thus leads to God.

Ghazālī mentions a love of beauty for its own sake, which is shared by all human beings. The beauty of nature is loved for itself alone, for its own pleasure. The love of greenery and water does not follow any other need than that of the mere enjoyment of nature. Beauty is also cherished because it frees people from sorrows, a concept that is very common in Arabic thought.

Among his statements on aesthetic beauty, Ghazālī speaks of the characteristic perfection which is related to a specific function or performance; a view that includes the notion of equilibrium.

> The beautiful horse is that which combines everything that is characteristic of a horse with regard to appearance, body color, beautiful movement and tractability; a beautiful writing combines everything that is characteristic of writing, such as harmony of letters, their correct relation to each other, right sequence and beautiful arrangement. The beauty of each object lies just in its characteristic perfection.[21]

Like the divine creation which reveals God's beauty, the work of human beings reflects their beauty: "The beautiful work of an author, the beautiful poem of a poet, the beautiful painting of a painter or the building of an architect reveal also the inner beauty of these men."[22]

Ghazālī adds that "pleasure is a form of cognition" (*al-ladhdha nawʿ idrāk*); "to enjoy is to know" (*man dhāqa ʿarifa*). Those who have no sense of pleasure are impassive and phlegmatic. God created beauty for humanity to perceive and enjoy in order to acquire a taste for the eternal bliss of the hereafter. People should be able to recognize the signs of God in his creation; if they fail to see the divine beyond worldly pleasures, they will be the victims of a delusion. It is up to them to decide to venerate the beauty of this world as a manifestation of God, or to regard it as an end in itself and remain blind to God. In spite of his allegiance to Ashʿarism which sees God as the absolute creator of all things and all actions, Ghazāī repeatedly emphasizes the freedom of choice. In his discourse on music, he does not follow early theologians such as Imām Shāfiʿī (d. 820) and Abū Ḥanīfa (d. 767) who condemned musical performances altogether, but he does discriminate between religious music and music performed in an illicit context, thus giving humankind the freedom and the responsibility to judge and choose between the permissible and the wrong.

Beauty is not only visual; it can be perceived by other senses as well. The senses of sight, smell, and touch, as well as cognition, have their own corresponding pleasures. There is a hierarchy in the perception of beauty: the more exalted the subject of our knowledge, the higher the pleasure. Ghazālī distinguishes between aesthetic and intelligible beauty. Only exoteric beauty is sensed through sight, hearing, touch, and taste, but there is also the beauty of abstract things such as knowledge and virtues, which is perceived by "inner sight" (*baṣīra bāṭina*). The beauty of virtues cannot be perceived by the senses.

> "The beauty of outer form which is seen with the bodily eye, can be experienced by children and animals, . . . whereas the beauty of the inward form can only be perceived by the eye of the heart, and the light of inner vision of man alone."

Inward vision is stronger than outward vision because the heart is more sensitive than the eye, and because the beauty perceived by the heart is more powerful than the beauty perceived by the eye. The beauty of proportion or pure color is perceived by sight, but the beauty of majesty, grandeur, superiority of character and goodness and all that is included in inner qualities is perceived by the sense of the heart.[23] Knowledge is an elevated form of pleasure and the perception of beauty. The knowledge of God is the perfect perception of beauty, for His beauty is perfect. The knowledge of Him is thus the utmost form of pleasure, surpassing all sensuous and intellectual satisfactions.

Despite his hostility toward philosophy, Ghazālī was influenced by Ibn Sīnā (d. 1063), who believed that pleasure seeking was deeply rooted in the human soul; all faculties of the soul have this feature in common. There is a qualitative difference between the various forms of pleasure reaching from the instinctive to the spiritual. The more people are able to abstract and discipline their speculative faculties, the closer they will come to the apprehension of exalted things and to the attainment of supreme happiness.[24]

Ghazālī thus qualifies the love of God as the highest form of beauty and the pursuit of pleasure. Pleasure is humankind's ultimate objective, and their love of beauty is linked to the pleasure it conveys. This is rooted in human nature. Human beings love themselves, their lives, and all that is good and pleasing to them. It is their basic love of self and their instinctive quest for pleasure that should lead them ultimately to God so that they may attain the supreme pleasure.[25] Love results from the similarity and harmony between the loving and the beloved; this justifies the human love of self, for humanity was created in God's image.

Ibn Qayyim al-Jawziyya (d. 1350), a key figure of anti-rationalist rigorist thought, distinguishes, as Ghazālī does, three types of pleasures: the first is a physical one, which humankind shares with animals and which includes basic needs; the second is produced by thought and imagination, which includes the search for greatness and power and is not shared by animals. The third is produced when mind and soul lead to the knowledge of God.[26] The yearning for perfection is the most powerful form of love. Love moves the universe; it is what drives the scholar to knowledge and the craftsman to his craft.[27]

THE SUFI WAY

Sharīʿa-oriented Islam is mainly concerned with religious practice in daily life; the sufis deal with the inner side of religion. Although the origins of sufism were connected with asceticism, the two should not be equated. It is characteristic of sufism, however, to emphasize the ephemeral and worthless character of this world and to preach detachment from worldly concerns in favor of the union with the Divine. The most radical ascetic mystic in Islam was an Arab woman named Rābiʿa al-ʿAdawiyya (d. 801), who said: "The contemplation of the Maker preoccupies me, so that I do not care to look upon what He has made."[28]

The most exuberant and passionate sufi figure was al-Ḥallāj (d. 922), whose search for the union with God assumed such extravagant proportions that he was accused of identifying himself with God and was executed for heresy, after severe torture. He remained, however, a symbol of the free form of religious devotion assumed by the sufis.[29]

Sufism in all its orientations identifies God and His creation with beauty and the veneration of God with the love of beauty. The beauty praised by the sufis is an inward beauty which is perceived by the "eye of the heart." The sufi aspires to lose himself in ecstasy (*fanāʾ*) in order to find God. This ecstasy can be reached through contemplation or through rituals, especially through the *samāʿ* or religious musical performances which also include dance.

Sufi literature is full of references to beauty, but it does not deal with mundane topics such as the meaning of the arts or the architecture of the mosque. When it deals with music or calligraphy, mystic literature is concerned solely with the individual's spiritual experience. The mystical approach to beauty is, because of its spirituality, *ipso facto* not aesthetic. An influence of mystic thought on Islamic arts, which some scholars have recently tried to demonstrate, cannot be supported by textual evidence. The evolution of Islamic art remained distinct from the emergence and the spread of sufism. In poetry, their principal medium, the sufis used traditional forms to express themselves, veiling their spiritual passion in the profane vocabulary of bacchic and erotic poetry.

The sufis describe their encounter with God in visual terms, using words such as gaze and vision. A favorite reference is a veil, or "veil of light," behind which God is concealed. The pioneer mystic al-Junayd of Baghdad (d. 910) wrote about his mystic experience:

> Though from my gaze profound
> Deep awe hath hid Thy face,
> In wondrous and ecstatic grace
> I feel Thee touch my inmost ground.[30]

The Egyptian mystic ʿUmar Ibn al-Fāriḍ (d. 1235) was the most important sufi poet of the Arab world; he was venerated as a saint even in his lifetime. About beauty he wrote:

> The beauty of every lovely thing that revealeth itself said unto me, "Take thy joy in me"; but I declared, "My purpose lieth beyond thee."[31]

> With my Beloved I alone have been
> When communings more sweet than evening airs
> Passed, and the Vision blest
> Was granted to my prayers,

That crowned me, else obscure, with endless fame,
The while amazed between
His beauty and His majesty
I stood in silent ecstasy,
Revealing that which o'er my spirit went and came.
Lo! in His face commingled
Is every charm and grace;
The whole of Beauty singled
Into a perfect face
Beholding Him would cry,
There is no God but He, and He is the most High![32]

The Neoplatonic doctrines of emanation, which had such an influence on Arabic philosophy, are manifest also in sufism, in the longing of the soul for the union with the One. The soul, attracted by divine beauty, is driven by a nostalgic movement toward its origins and the origins of the universe. Like the philosophers who thought that the quest for knowledge leads to happiness in this world, the sufis also believed that the soul can reach its goal in this life by achieving individual union with God. For the jurists and theologians, however, supreme happiness is not to be attained in this life, but in paradise.[33]

The Ikhwān al-Ṣafā, or Brethren of Purity, were a group of five scholars who lived in 10th-century Basra and wrote esoteric philosophical epistles. Their philosophy combined Greek thought of Neoplatonic and Neopythagorean forms with Shīʿa ideas. Although their philosophy was inspired by mathematics—"the science of numbers is the root of other sciences, the fount of wisdom, the starting point of all knowledge, and the origin of all concepts"[34]—they did not apply them to formulate aesthetic concepts, but referred to them only in a metaphysical, philosophical context.

In the view of the Ikhwān al-Ṣafā this world is a temporary reflection of the spiritual and eternal world; the human body is "an adorned figure" which is only a reflection of the perfect soul. Humanity should free itself from the illusory worldly desires whose satisfaction can only be ephemeral and aspire to the higher eternal realm of the soul.[35] Absolute beauty is an attribute of God, and the hierarchy of being is dependent upon the degree to which anything possesses beauty or participates in the Beauty of God.

> He made these His works manifest, to the end that the intelligent might contemplate them; and He brought into view all that was in His invisible world, that the observant might behold it and acknowledge His skill and peerlessness and omnipotence and soleness, and not stand in need of proof and demonstration. Further, these forms, which are perceived in the material world, are the similitudes of those which exist in the world of spirits save that the latter are composed of light and are subtle; whereas the former are dark and dense. And, as a picture corresponds in every limb with the animal it presents, so these forms, too, correspond with those which are found in the spiritual world. But these are the movers, and those are the moved . . . The forms which exist in the other world endure; whereas these perish and pass away.[36]

> Know that the perfect manufacturing of an object indicates the existence of a wise and perfect artisan even when he is veiled and inaccessible to sense perception. He who meditates upon botanical objects will of necessity know that the things of his reign issue from a perfect artisan.[37]

Ibn Ṭufayl (d. 1185/6) is the author of a Neoplatonic allegorical novel called *Ḥayy Ibn Yaqẓān* (The Living Son of the Wakeful), a symbolic name invented earlier by Ibn Sīnā to designate the active intellect (*ʿaql faʿʿāl*) a supernatural, but not divine, power which assists the soul in its search for supreme knowledge.[38] For Ibn Ṭufayl man can attain knowledge without any outside agent; he only needs his own reason. His novel tells of a man generated spontaneously, who lives solitary on a desert island, nursed by a deer. Ḥayy was able, through various stages of contemplation, to reach knowledge and wisdom until his soul achieved the contemplation of God. In the second part of the novel, he encounters human society whose religious worship according to scripture disappointed him. His was the way of spiritual illumination, not of religious law. Ḥayy discovers God's "workmanship" through contemplation of the world, its beauty and perfection. Looking at God's creation made him long for the Creator. Having recognized His beauty, he began to enquire about the apprehensive faculties that led him to this knowledge, and found that it was his soul alone. In this narrative Ibn Ṭufayl presented visual beauty as the highest form of beauty that can be perceived by the physical senses—sight being considered in ancient philosophy as the highest of all senses. He concluded that the ultimate encounter of the soul with the Supreme Being, once it has freed itself from the corporeal, is essentially a matter of eternal vision and delight. Ibn Ṭufayl's aim was to show that illuminative wisdom can be attained by mysticism, through the annihilation of the self and its absorption in God. What philosophers seek through speculative rational thinking, the mystic pursues in his solitude.[39]

Ibn ʿArabī (d. 1240) was one of the boldest figures of Islamic mysticism. His sufi approach, with its Neoplatonic orientation, was unorthodox and controversial; its impact was particularly pronounced in eastern Islam and in Turkey. He saw the world as consisting of a visible exoteric and an invisible part. The visible physical world mirrors the invisible. God is the invisible world and He is reflected through His creation in the visible world. Following Platonic concepts, according to which love is the prime mover of all things toward the beautiful and the eternally perfect, he conceived beauty as the cause of all love. One loves God because He is beautiful, and He loves us and all His creation because He loves beauty. He is Himself the lovable lover and beloved and thus the origin and the end of the cosmos. God's beauty is the source of all beauty, the physical, spiritual, and intellectual.[40] He should be worshipped through all forms of beauty including the temporal one. Beauty is powerful and attracts love and desire; the sympathy between humanity and the universe is based upon love (*ʿishq*).

Ibn ʿArabī's esoteric discourse on beauty is not aesthetic. Beauty is theophany—a manifestation of God—and mystic love is the religion of beauty.[41] If one loves someone for his or her beauty it is God's beauty that one loves, since God created the human being in His own image. Humanity is the visible manifestation of divinity and the world is a mirror of His beauty. Beauty is the generator of divine love because God is eternal beauty. He loves His creatures and by doing so He loves Himself.

Through the mystical experience the soul finds its unity with the whole. In this form of mystic love, the contemplation of human beauty is included as a sacral phenomenon which reaches beyond the object contemplated, fulfilling the unity of the sensuous with the spiritual.[42] The sufi worshiper is passionate to the extent of being lost in the love of God. The encounter with perfect beauty and the intimacy with Him (*uns*) is a source of supreme pleasure and satisfaction (*riḍā*).

The terms *uns* and *riḍā* were criticized by the orthodox for their sensual associations, but Ghazālī refuted such arguments as superficial.[43]

According to Nicholson, "The devotional and mystical love of God developed into ecstasy and enthusiasm which finds in the sensuous imagery of human love the most suggestive medium for its expression."[44] Ibn ʿArabī and other sufis used an erotic ambiguous poetry to express their love of God. Composed in the traditional forms of *ghazal* (love poetry) or *khamriyya* (bacchic poetry), it leaves the choice to the listener or reader whether to stop at the literal meaning or to look through this veil into deeper religious passion. The Arab sufis thus did not create a new artistic language of their own, but adopted instead the established literary traditions, toying with ambiguity and symbolism.

> Oh, her beauty—the tender maid! Its brilliance gives light like lamps to one travelling in the dark.
> She is a pearl hidden in a shell of hair as black as jet,
> A pearl for which Thought dives and rema
> ins unceasingly in the deeps of that ocean.
> He who looks upon her deems her to be a gazelle of the sand-hills, because of her shapely neck and the loveliness of her gestures.[45]

The symbolism of love and wine poetry was meant to convey the individual mystic experience, which is otherwise difficult to transmit. Using the medium of traditional bacchic poetry to symbolize rapture and ecstasy, ʿUmar Ibn al-Fāriḍ (1181–1235) wrote:

> We drank in memory of the beloved
> a wine
> we were drunk with it
> before the creation of the vine.[46]

Because Ibn ʿArabī's philosophy of metaphysical beauty included temporal beauty in the mystic experience, it was controversial and refuted by many theologians. Commenting on and criticizing the sufis who contemplate temporal beauty in search of God's manifestation, they warned against the evil role that the eye, as an instrument of temptation and sin, can play. As repeatedly formulated by Ibn Qayyim al-Jawziyya, an outspoken opponent of Ibn ʿArabī's school, physical beauty can ravish the heart, taking it away from God toward sin. He speaks of *idmān al-naẓar,* which means "addiction of gaze," implying mainly erotic seduction.

Because the eye is the "mirror" of the heart, it can generate greed and sin.[47]

Muslim society attaches enormous importance to sight in the relationship between the sexes, which explains the prohibition against free women revealing their faces to male strangers. Aside from the erotic aspect, gaze is equated with desire altogether, and the eye can be evil. Through the eye desire is aroused, which can generate envy; it then becomes the evil eye. Everything beautiful is liable to be hit by the evil eye and is thus vulnerable. It is wise to avoid the evil eye by not showing one's blessings. When something is *manẓūr* (viewed), it has been hit by the evil eye, and itself becomes a source of bad luck.

THE SYMBOLISM OF LIGHT

Light is a central motif in Neoplatonism and in sufism. Through the mediation of Islamic philosophy, light metaphysics came to play a paramount role in medieval Christian theology and concepts of beauty. Beauty was equated with light. In Islam light is the symbol of wisdom and knowledge; it is also a central symbol in sufism. The source of this symbolism is in the Koran:

> God is the light of heavens and of the earth; His light is like a niche in which there is a lamp; the lamp is in a glass and the glass is like a shining star; it is lit from a blessed tree, an olive-tree, neither an eastern nor a western one; its oil almost shines alone even if no fire touches it; light upon light. God leads to His light whom He will, and God creates allegories for man, and God knows all things. (24:35)

A number of other verses in the Holy Book also refer to light as the symbol of God's revelation, of knowledge and wisdom. The Koran brought light to the believers on earth. "The earth will shine with the light of her Lord and the Book will be laid open." (39:69) Scriptures are "light-giving books" (*kitāb munīr*) (3:184; 22:8; 35:25).

> Believe in God and His apostle, and in the light which We have revealed. (64:8)

> We have sent you down a glorious light. (4:174)

God leads humanity to the light of His revelation (5:15; 33:46), which is an emanation of His own light; it is the guidance of the sufi.

For Ghazālī all things are a reflection of the divine light. He mentions light also in another, subjective, meaning, that of the inward sight (*al-baṣīra al-bāṭina*), which is the light of faith and the faculty of discerning the truth. Like the theologians, the philosophers equated light with reason because it frees man from darkness. Reason is light because it makes things manifest and light is primarily an attribute of God.

The Muslim doctrine of light was strongly inspired by Zoroastrianism and Hellenistic gnosticism. Ibn Sīnā referred to beauty and light to define the movement of the soul toward the Supreme Being. When the soul has freed itself from the bondage of the body, it becomes unified with the light of the absolute good and beautiful. It acquires a wisdom that invites the earthbound soul to turn away from the crude pleasure of the body and to fix its gaze upon the ultimate source of beauty and light. The dazzling brilliance of this supreme source of light dazzles the vision, like the sun, "which is amply manifest only when it sets."[48]

According to Ibn Sīnā, God is the source of the overflowing light which fills all things. In a series of symbolic narratives belonging to his Oriental philosophy, the philosopher describes the journey of the soul toward the light of wisdom, guided by an angelic or metaphysical companion, the active intellect. In Ibn Sīnā's symbolic narrative called Ḥayy Ibn Yaqẓān (the Living Son of the Wakeful),[49] the soul, seeking the encounter of the Wise and Beautiful, meets the metaphysical guide who is Ḥayy b. Yaqẓān. Ḥayy travels across the world, with his face turned to his Father, the Wakeful, the source of all wisdom and light. With his help, the soul penetrates new regions of the metaphysical universe between the corruptible matter and the immaterial Orient that is the origin of the light that all forms, whether material or intelligible, bear.

Suhrawardī (d. 1191) took over the illuminationist ideas of Ibn Sīnā and developed a philosophy of enlightenment based on the Divine Light as the very substance of the universe. His metaphysical vision was that of a world where the east symbolized the rising light and the west was darkness and exile. The universe itself consisted of a complex system of lights, with light and darkness, or spirit and matter, ruled by immaterial lights. God guides the entire universe toward His light. In this universe the soul, in its occidental exile, has to free itself from the prison of the body, which is darkness, starting the journey to the east, from matter into light, from the lower to the higher spheres of the universe.

For the Aristotelian Ibn Rushd (d. 1198) God is light; just as light makes colors visible, without being itself visible, God is the source of all sensible experience but is nevertheless enveloped in veils of light.[50]

About his apprehension of the divine light, ʿUmar Ibn al-Fāriḍ said:

. . . . From his light
The lantern of my essence shone on me;
My eve in me was radiant as my morn.
And I was made to see myself, myself
Yet here; and I was he; and I beheld
That he was I, that light my radiance.[51]

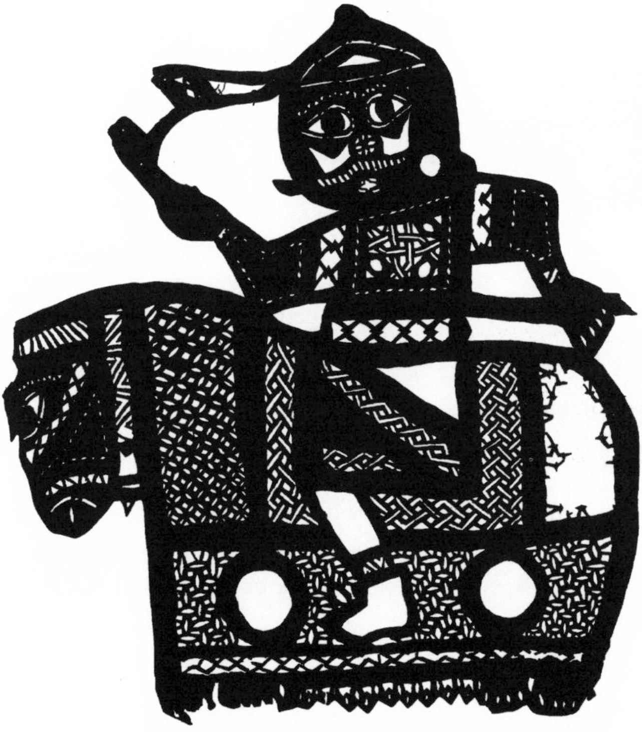

Shadow-play figure, Egypt, 15th century. Deutsches Ledermuseum, Offenbach.
Archive Doris Behrens-Abouseif.

Ibn ʿArabī viewed light as everything through which apprehension takes place: "If you apprehend sound, you call the apprehending Light hearing, and if you perceive by hearing, you call it seeing."[52]

In accordance with the mystic's interpretation of the visible world as the shadow of the spiritual and luminous world,[53] the shadow play has been repeatedly used since the 10th century as the symbol of humanity's existence in this world. The world is a theater, the figures are moved by one invisible hand; they are shadows that come and go behind a veil. They all vanish; the mover remains.[54] Among the sufis particularly attracted by this Platonic image was ʿUmar Ibn al-Fāriḍ. He composed a poem describing the shadow play spectacle in interesting detail, with birds singing in trees, camels travelling across deserts and ships across seas, horsemen and footsoldiers involved in hunts or battles, hunting scenes between birds and animals of prey, sea monsters pursuing ships. The spectator follows the events, in grief or enjoyment, weeping and laughing alternately.

> And thou shalt find all that appears to thee
> And whatsoever thou dost contemplate
> The acts of one alone, but in the veils
> Of occultation wrapt: when he removes
> The curtain, thou beholdest none but him
> . . . .

The mystic goes on to use the image of the veil in another variant:

> So in its acts my soul resembles him;
> My sense is like the figures; and my screen
> The body's vesture. . . .[55]

The veil in sufism is a corollary to the theme of light. A series of veils conceal God's face from humanity, their luminosity varying according to their closeness to the divine. The closer one comes to the truth, the more translucent the veil will be.

Secular Beauty and Love

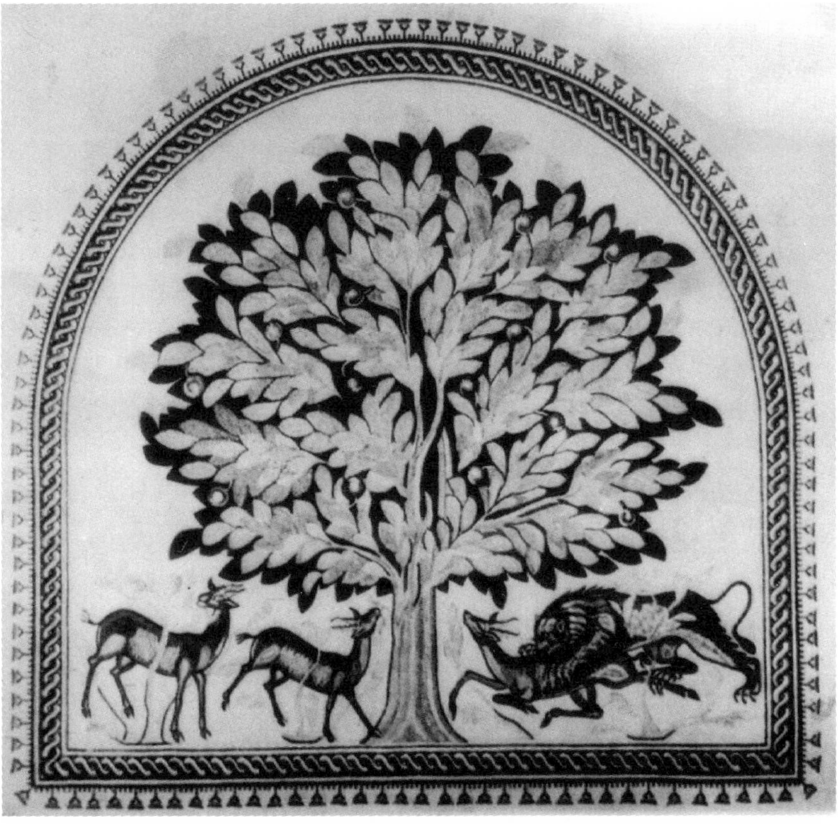

Mosaic at Khirbat al-Mafjar, Umayyad "desert palace"

Proportion, Harmony, and the Psychological Factor

The Arabs inherited from the Greeks the doctrine that proportion was the basis of beauty. This principle was adopted in all periods and in the context of various disciplines, in particular in the arts of calligraphy and music. The doctrine of the harmony of proportion allowed the formulation of universal aesthetic statements applicable to all arts as well as to human beauty. In the Ikhwān al-Ṣafā's concept of beauty, based on Pythagorean ideas of mathematical proportions, the same principle of the proportionality of elements defines the beauty of calligraphy, music, painting, and sculpture, the efficiency of a medicine, the taste of food, and the goodness of a character.[56] They considered geometry as the basis of all sciences because it established a relationship between the positions of objects, and it allowed the mind to think in abstract terms, thus leading to its exaltation and purification.[57] The Ikhwān al-Ṣafā also adopted the Pythagorean notions of arithmetical and geometrical relationship as basic to the harmony pervading the universe.[58] Most Arabic thinkers, however, defined harmony as the optimal proportions that make something beautiful.

Bīrūnī (d. 1048) counted poetry and music among the mathematical sciences, emphasizing their effect on the soul, which loves harmonious mathematical compositions.[59]

Al-Jāḥiẓ (d. 869) valued equilibrium as the basis of all forms of beauty: all that exceeds the limits of its own characteristics, whether it is a physical object or something abstract, violates the rules of beauty. Equilibrium is vital to the beauty of the soul as well as the body. It is valid for the arts of architecture, carpet weaving, textile weaving, and even for canals, a view that recalls modern concepts of art and industrial design.[60] The principle of equilibrium endorsed by Jāḥiẓ conforms with the refined society in which he lived, which created the *adab* culture (which will be discussed below).

In the 12th century ʿAbd al-Laṭīf al-Baghdādī, physician and scholar, praised the beauty of the Sphinx of Giza for its harmonious proportions;[61] the role of proportions in human beauty was also acknowledged by Ibn Qayyim al-Jawziyya in the 14th century.[62]

The concept of harmony as the universal criterion for beauty was confirmed by the literary theorist ʿAbd al-Qāhir al-Jurjānī (d. 1078), who used the example of a piece of jewelry, a ring or an earring, that acquires its beauty through the harmonious composition of its elements. His notion of harmonious composition, however, included also dissimilar elements, for beauty is achieved with contrast, which he calls "the affinity of contraries" (*shiddat iʾtilāf fī shiddat ikhtilāf*).[63] He wrote further:

> This (harmony of composition) is manifest in all crafts and artistic activities which are associated with subtlety, fineness and skill. In the images produced in such crafts it is always the case that the more widely different in shape and appearance their parts are and the more perfect the harmony achieved between these parts, the more fascination the images will possess and the more deserving the praise for their skills of their creators.[64]

Ibn Khaldūn's most explicit statement on beauty says that visible and audible beauty "harmonizes with the cognitive soul, which enjoys perceiving that which is in harmony with itself" (*munāsib li'l-nafs al-mudrika fataltadhdhu bi idrāki mulāʾimihā*), in the same manner as "lovers' souls meet each other and blend." The enjoyment of perfumes belongs to this type of affinity. He adds that the "perfection of proportion and setting are the quintessence of beauty in everything" (*kamāl al-munāsaba wa'l-waḍʿ wa dhalika huwa maʿnā al-jamāl wa'l-ḥusn fī kulli madrak*).[65]

Ibn Khaldūn's idea of harmony includes both the harmonious composition of the object and the affinity generated between the object and the subject. The criteria of proportion and harmony remained flexible and subjective; they were not tied to objective universal criteria, as in Greek culture where they were applied and related to the visual arts. The appreciation of proportion and harmony that was decisive in the art of calligraphy, for example, did not hinder the general rather atomistic approach to poetry which emphasized the autonomy of the verse rather than the form of the poem as a whole. When Baghdādī speaks of the Sphinx, Jāḥiẓ of female beauty, and Jurjānī of the elegant ring, none of them refers to a canon or exact criteria comparable to those set for calligraphy to qualify the beauty of their objects. It is rather their subjective perceptions—the pleasing and psychological effect produced by the objects—that determine the beauty they recognize. Harmony is often understood as the affinity between the object and its beholder. The psychological factor has always been emphasized as fundamental and universal in the aesthetic experience. The articulation of the psychological factor in the perception of beauty goes back to Ibn al-Haytham, known in the West as Alhazen (935–1038/9).

Ibn al-Haytham was neither philosopher nor theologian, but a physicist and mathematician. He achieved a breakthrough in the field of optics by distinguishing between the physical and the mental aspects of perception. To see an object is not just a visual process, but a complex process that includes mental mechanisms. The perception of the external world is achieved when the mind interprets the visual sensations that reach the eye mechanically. Sight perceives various properties in an object which, either individually or in conjunction with one another, produce beauty which has a pleasing effect on the soul. The properties of the object do not produce beauty in all situations but in some rather than others. Proportionality is one of these properties. Sight perceives only the manifest features of the object without analyzing them; it is the mental faculty of discriminating through analogies that perceives beauty.[66] The perception of beauty is thus based on an intellectual process involving the ability to judge, or distinguish objectively, making use of memory. We recognize shapes through their similarity to images in our mind. In perceiving we compare things and discriminate between them, recording the differences and similarities. The process of judgment leads the "raw material" perceived by the eye to the mind which sorts it, categorizes it, and elaborates on it by associating it with other things, leading it then to the heart.

There is a striking parallel between Ibn al-Haytham's analysis of the mental process of vision and the theory of perception formulated by his contemporary Ibn Sīnā with which he must have been acquainted. This theory explains the ability of the mind to absorb and integrate objects perceived by the senses by translating them into the abstract medium of images in the brain; in a subsequent procedure these images are submitted to analysis and judgment, acquiring their meaning after being associated and compared to other impressions already registered in memory. The subsequent mental act produces abstract and conceptual thinking. By combining Ibn al-Haytham's with Ibn Sīnā's concepts, the perception of beauty appears as the product of man's faculty of abstract thinking based on his sensuous perceptions. Beauty is thus not "ontological," to use Grassi's term.

> Position produces beauty, and many things that look beautiful do so only because of order and position . . . Similarly, composition, even though many forms of visible objects are felt to be beautiful and appealing only because of the composition and order of their parts among themselves.[67]

Although his work belongs to the field of optics and the psychology of seeing, Ibn Haytham's ideas show a pronounced aesthetic sensitivity; he was in fact the first to make a psychological analysis of visual aesthetics. His scientific impact was of great importance both in Islam and in the West where his ideas were propagated by the Polish philosopher Witelo.[68] His theory of aesthetic, however, did not lead to a far-reaching conceptualization of this subject, but remained rather exceptional in Arabic tradition.

Ibn al-Haytham lists several types of beauty: ". . .some have as their cause one of the particular properties in the form; others are caused by a number of the particular properties in the form; still others are caused by a conjunction of the properties one with another, and not by the properties themselves; and the cause of still others is composed of the properties in their harmony."[69] Among the properties that produce beauty, in the sense that "they produce in the soul an effect such that the form appears beautiful," Ibn al-Haytham enumerates light, colors, distance (the stars in the sky), position (letters in calligraphy), solidity (human and animal bodies), shape, size, separateness (flowers scattered in a meadow), continuity, number (stars in the sky), motion (dance), rest, profile (jewelry), smoothness (cloth, utensils), transparency (precious stones), opacity (colors and shapes), shadow, darkness (like the beauty of lamps), similarity (paired organs in a body), and variation and change within the same body (thickness of a nose or the letters of a script). None of these properties produces beauty in all situations; it is the combination of these properties with one another that generated most of the beauty perceived by the sense of sight.

The idea that beauty is a combination of factors was often expressed. The aesthetic experience is viewed as the result of the quality of the object and the perspective of the subject, and is thus contrary to aesthetic dogmas that postulate specific fixed rules in the qualification of beauty. This approach conforms with an established tendency to relativism, according to which bad and good are not absolute values, but a matter of circumstances and subjective experience. Jāḥiẓ was the initiator of a literary genre dealing with contraries, or merits and faults in the same thing. He sets out to demonstrate that reality had simultaneously a positive and a negative side; it was the quality and proportion of the mixture and its impact on the human mind that produced its value.[70] He similarly viewed the human being as a microcosm that combines all elements and attributes that exist in nature, with all their disparity and contradictions.[71]

Since the perception of beauty is based on a mental process, it requires intellectual skill for its accomplishment. For Jāḥiẓ, "the subject of beauty is too subtle and too delicate to be perceived by just anybody; this also applies to abstract things. Judgment can be articulated only by one who is able to see deeply, whose eyes can communicate their perception to the heart, for only then can the mind articulate a judgment."[72]

Whether because of his direct influence or a general attitude, Ibn al-Haytham's emphasis on the psychological factor is endorsed in most Arabic statements on beauty. Ghazālī recognized an emotional type of perception emphasizing the role of sympathy which disregards formal criteria and follows the affinity of the soul (*tanāsub al-arwāḥ*).[73]

Ibn Sīnā conceived pleasure as dependent on two factors, perfection and the perception of it. The latter was a form of knowledge and thus variable and relative. The intensity of pleasure is proportional to the degree of perfection and the extent of its perception.[74]

Referring to poetry, Jurjānī, who dealt thoroughly with the psychological roots of its aesthetic effect, wrote:

> Human nature is so created, and human instinctive and innate qualities are such, that when something appears whence it is not usually expected to appear, and when it emerges from a source which is not its normal one, the soul feels deeper fondness of, and greater affection for it. It is as exciting

and amazing to reveal the existence of something in a place in which it is not known to belong, as it is to create something which does not exist at all, or whose very existence is not realized.[75]

An episode reported in the *Book of Songs* (*al-Aghānī*) by Iṣbahānī (d. 967) illustrates the emotional factor in the perception of beauty. During a visit to Constantinople, an Arab heard in the street a voice singing an Arabic song. He was delighted by what he heard, but then he asked himself whether this delight was due to the quality of the performance or to the thrill of hearing an Arabic song in Constantinople.[76] When the 9th-century poet al-Mutanabbī wrote

The radiant stars with beauty strike our eyes
Because midst gloom opaque we see them rise[77]

he was interpreting beauty in lyrical terms, but also, like Ibn al-Haytham, as relative to the surrounding conditions and in combination with the faculty of judgment. The awareness of the psychological moment is thus deeply rooted in Arabic culture. It had a strong impact on European thought, in particular on Thomas of York, who used Arabic sources to emphasize the psychological and subjective character of beauty.[78]

The inclusion of the emotional factor is significant because it leads necessarily to pleasure as decisive for the qualification of beauty and for the aesthetic experience.[79] The concept of beauty as a matter of emotional and subjective perception rather than of objective criteria indicates the separation between the beautiful-and-pleasing and the morally good, i.e., the aesthetic approach to beauty.

The only universal principle that governed beauty in Arabic culture was its association with pleasure. But pleasure has many sources which can reach the heart in many ways; it is a blend of factors which address various senses and perceptions. De Bruyne cites Roger Bacon as having been under Arab influence when he defined the full aesthetic pleasure as the simultaneous satisfaction of all the senses.[80] Muslim theologians and philosophers distinguished various categories of pleasure depending on the qualities of the instincts and desires they satisfied and on the excellence of their objects, reaching from the appetitive to the abstract. In his study of Aristotle, Abū Naṣr al-Farābī (d. 950) distinguished two types of cognition, one that is useful and another that is good in itself, for its mere pleasure. Moreover, he attributed delectable things and their corresponding pleasures to different categories according to their physical or intellectual natures.

> They [men] desire sensible things, the apprehension of which by sense-perception is not useful to them in any one of those four things[81]—for instance, statues, elegant sceneries, objects delightful to hear and to smell, and objects pleasurable to touch—for nothing else besides having them as pleasurable objects of sense-perception. For "pleasurable" means nothing other than that one is apprehending most excellently a most excellent object of apprehension; for there cannot be pleasure without apprehension; it is present in [animals] that apprehend by sense-perception and absent from those that do not. Likewise, there are, besides the knowledge of sensible things, other cognitions obtained by sense-perception that man may desire although he confines himself to knowing and apprehending and to the pleasure he experiences in apprehending them: for instance, the myths, stories, histories of peoples, and histories of nations, that man narrates and to which he listens solely for the delight they give. (For to delight in something means nothing other than the achievement of comfort and pleasure).[82]

Nature and Artifice

The enjoyment of beauty, Ghazālī writes, dissipates sorrows. The Arabs believed in the psychosomatic effect of beauty, without distinguishing between beauty that was natural and beauty that was man-made. Beauty as such, whose nature is manifold and complex, was believed to have a soothing and healing effect on the body and the spirit. Poetry was enjoyed accompanied by music and wine, all three helping to avert unpleasant feelings. Some medical books recommend that the *ḥammām*, the temple of hygiene par excellence, should be decorated with paintings because images can substitute for nature in conveying a soothing effect on man.

The Koranic descriptions of paradise, where art mingles with natural landscape, exemplify the Arab approach to beauty and pleasure. The inhabitants of paradise are richly dressed and adorned with jewelry, they dwell in palaces and pavilions made of pearls and set amidst trees, valleys and streams. A cool breeze and scent fill the air. They have intercourse with women of eternal youth, and enjoy banquets served in golden dishes with drinks from silver vessels.[83] The *ḥadīth* texts devoted to paradise elaborate on the Koranic descriptions, adding more items to its delights, such as music.

Even an intellectual like Abū 'l-ʿAlāʾ al-Maʿarrī (d. 1057/8), one of the greatest Arab poets and a freethinker, imagined paradise not in abstract terms as did Dante, but as an Islamic paradise with all its carnal delights. In his version it is an abode of poets and thinkers. In his *Risālat al-Ghufrān* (*Epistle of Forgiveness*) Abū 'l-ʿAlāʾ imagines his friend Ibn al-Qāriḥ, not without irony, as having died and reached paradise. There, he finds the heavenly garden to be a kind of salon where poets and freethinkers meet to discuss poems and ideas, like "literary bohemians" as Nicholson put it, rather than a meeting place of the pious and virtuous. Unlike Dante's Paradiso, it is a voluptuous place where humans and animals are compensated for their worldly sufferings with all the earthly pleasures promised in the Koran such as banquets with music, dance, hunt

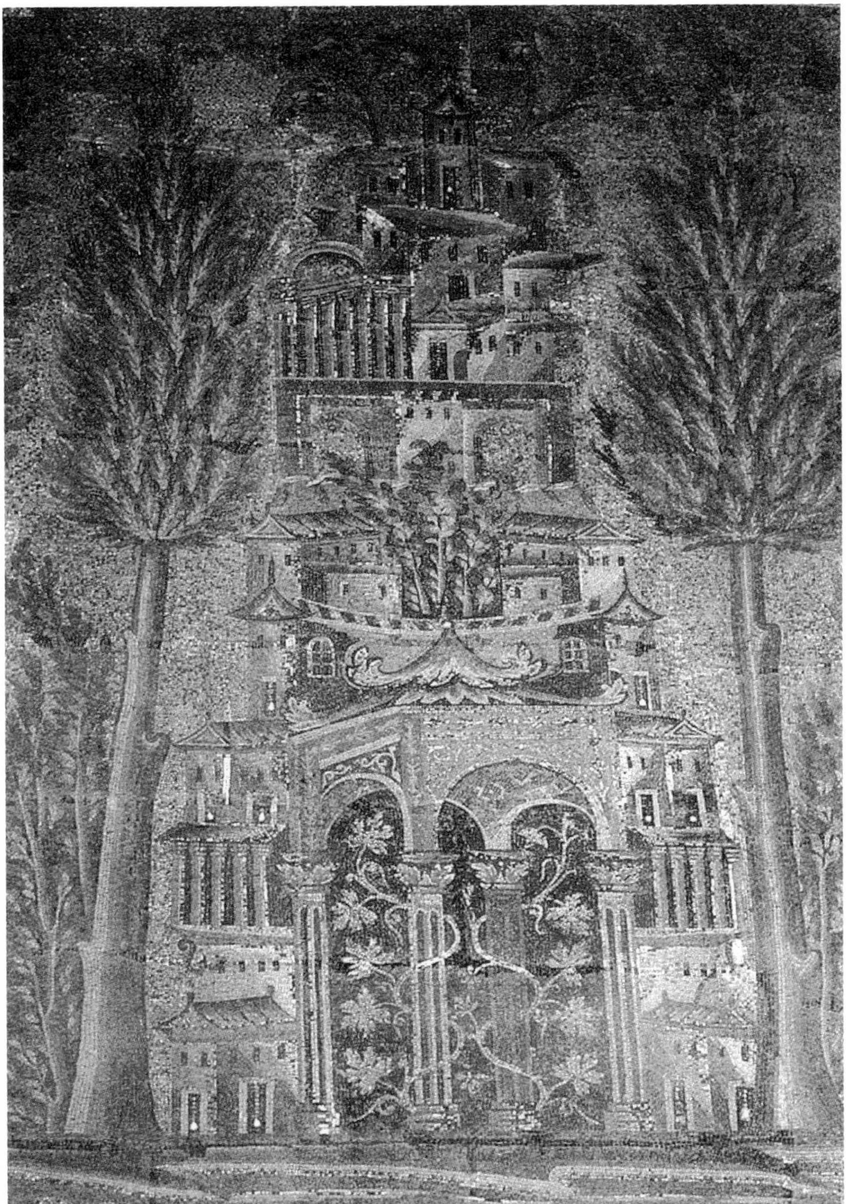

Mosaic from the Great Mosque of Damascus, early 8th century.
Archive Doris Behrens-Abouseif.

and, of course, sex.[84]

The landscape of paradise is not wild pure nature, but rather embellished and ornamented with artistic and luxurious objects, like those made by artists on earth. The arts of jewelry, metalwork, textiles, and architecture, all of which had a prominent place in Arabic Islamic culture, are represented in paradise, as God's creation to gratify its inhabitants.

Paradise is a garden, and a garden can be a small paradise. The word *junayna* (garden) is the diminutive of *janna*, which is a word for paradise. Like paradise, the gardens of the Muslim world cannot be imagined without design or without architectural adornments to enhance the landscape; their function is always associated with sensuous pleasures. The perception of nature in Arabic poetry was mostly linked to love and bacchic pastimes. Several poetic genres, the *zahriyyāt*, *rawḍiyyāt*, and *rabīʿiyyāt* (flower, garden, and spring poems, respectively), celebrated nature. Flowers were compared with gems and with details of the female body, and sometimes vice-versa. The poet Ibn al-Rūmī (d. 896) compares nature in spring with a woman who has adorned herself to meet her lover.

This combination of natural and artificial elements characterizes the decoration of the first great Islamic monuments, the Dome of the Rock in Jerusalem (691) and the Great Mosque of Damascus (706). In the first, plants and trees are adorned with jewels, and in the second, landscape is adorned with architecture. In both imageries, natural and man-made artistic beauty are integrated. Although the individual patterns are of Byzantine or other origins, the thematic blend presented in these mosaics already displays Arabic taste and aesthetics, as expressed in the visual arts and in poetry. It shows the "nonrealistic use of realistic shapes and anti-naturalistic combination of natural forms," as Ettinghausen and Grabar write in their introduction to Islamic art.[85] It reveals the same principle behind the arabesque, which is the synthetization of a vegetal motif, transcending nature with artifice and fantasy.

The Palace of the Tree built by the caliph al-Muqtadir (d. 932) in Baghdad had a pond in the center of which was a silver tree with gilt silver singing birds. On both sides of the pond were mechanical statues of mounted horsemen who could appear to be fighting each other. There was also a smaller pond of mercury on which gilt boats floated. It was in the middle of a garden that included a zoo with (real) wild animals, among them a hundred lions.[86] A description of the 9th-century garden of Egypt's Tulunid ruler Khumārawayh has a similar blend of natural and artistic elements, with trees clad in copper sheets and flowerbeds shaped like inscription bands. A pool of mercury reflected the moonlight.

Arabic poetry is full of metaphors where jewelry, flowers, and brocades intermingle. Describing the narcissus, the poet al-Ṣanawbarī wrote:

> Pearls unfolding from yellow sapphires (which rest) on emerald stems over carpets of fine sundus-silk.[87]

Abū Nuwās (d. ca. 810), the most famous bacchic poet in the Arabic language, praises ruby-red wine and a view of multicolored gardens as means of banishing sorrows:

> Behold the clouds embroidering
> with dewy fingers the earthy gown with fragrant flowers,
> lilies of the valley fresh to be plucked, lavender,
> violets and red anemones,
> a harvest of roses dazzling
> as suns rising amidst the twigs,
> in red, white and yellow
> and all splendid colors
> like necklaces of rubies and pearls
> with beads of gold
> set between olivines,
> a shining string along the garden.[88]

The following page of the *Arabian Nights*, from a 14th-century text, gives another vivid example of this aesthetic blend:

> When we had our fill of such delicious food and fine drink, they brought to us two gilded basins, and we washed our hands. Then they brought incense, with which we perfumed ourselves. Then they brought rosewater scented with musk in bowls of gilded crystal, encircled with carved figures of camphor and ambergris and set with all kinds of jewels, and after we scented ourselves, we returned to our couches.
>
> Then the maid asked us to rise and we rose and she led us to another chamber. When she opened the door, we found ourselves in a room covered with a silk carpet, under a dome that rested on a hundred pillars, at the base of each of which stood a bird or a beast dipped in gold. We sat and

began to admire the carpet, which, with its gold ground and patterns of white and red roses, repeated the colors and patterns of the dome.

In the room, resting on tables, there were more than a hundred trays of crystal and gold, set with all kinds of jewels. At the upper end of the room, numerous lovely couches, covered with fabrics of various colors, stood, each before an arched window that opened on a garden.

The garden looked as if it had the same carpet for a floor cover. There the water flowed from a large pond to a smaller one surrounded by sweet basil, lilies, and narcissus in pots of inlaid gold. The thickly intertwined branches were heavy with ripe fruits, so that whenever the windy host passed through them, the fruits dropped on the water, while birds of all kinds swooped down after them, clapping their wings and singing.

To the right and left of the pond stood couches of sandalwood covered with silver, and on each couch reclined a damsel more dazzling than the sun, wearing a gorgeous dress and holding a lute or some other musical instrument to her bosom. The damsels' music blended with the cooing of the birds, and the wafting wind joined the rippling water, as the breeze blew, lifting a rose here and downing a fruit there.

With dazzled eyes and minds, we contemplated such great means and reflected on such abundant blessings and, turning from the garden with the pond to the room with the dome, we enjoyed the loveliness of the garden, the gracefulness of the art, and the magnificence of the endeavor and marveled at the grandeur of the sight and beauty of the scene.[89]

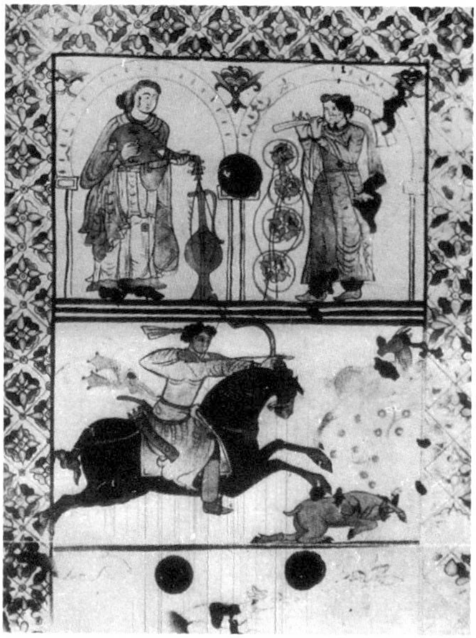

Musicians and hunting scene from Umayyad desert palace

Here carpets with flower patterns, natural flowers, gold and crystal, the singing of the birds and the music of the lute, the breeze and the incense, the hall and the garden, all mingle to produce the right mixture to ravish the senses. This description did not spring out of the narrator's imagination; rather it

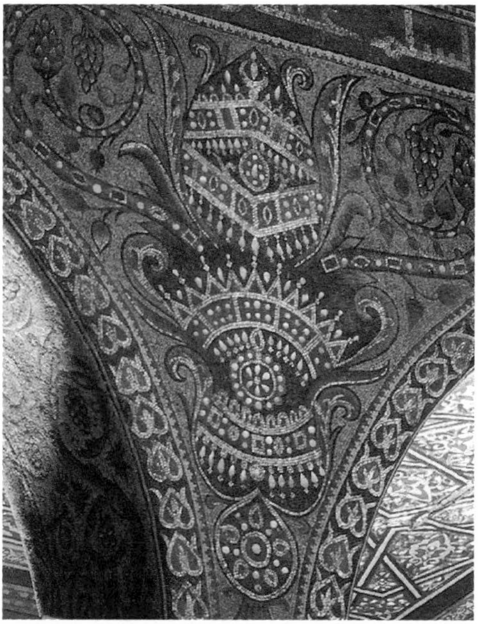

Mosaic ornament, Dome of the Rock, Jerusalem, late 7th c.

conformed to the accounts given in Arabic literary sources of the gatherings given by the caliphs of the Omayyad and Abbasid periods for poetic and musical performances. An exquisite setting, elegant garments, food and wine, perfumes and scents, music and poetry performed by artists contributed to convey delight. It is the ideal which the Koranic paradise promises.

The following passage from the *Arabian Nights* also shows the soothing powers of aesthetic blends of architecture, birds, lamps, and scents. The narrator is invited to dwell in a palace with a hundred rooms, of which he is allowed to open only ninety-nine. He moves from one room to another, enjoying the contents of each.

> Then I opened a third door and found myself in a large hall covered with all kinds of colored marble, rare metals, and precious stones and hung with cages of aloe- and sandalwood, full of all kinds of singing birds, such as nightingales, thrushes, pigeons, ringdoves, turtledoves, silver doves and Nubian doves. There I enjoyed myself, felt happy, and forgot my cares.[90]

In another room:

> I found the floor strewn with saffron and saw lamps of gold and silver, fed with costly oils, and saw fragrant candles burning with aloes and ambergris. I also saw two incense burners, each as large as a kneading bowl, full of glowing embers in which burned the incense of aloewood, ambergris, musk, and frankincense, and as the incense burned, the smoke rose to blend with the odors of the candles and the saffron, filling the chamber with perfume.[91]

The love of elegant settings had been pursued to excess in Arab court life of the classical period. There is the case of an Abbasid caliph who gave audience in a hall covered with pink tapestry opening on a garden whose trees had pink flowers, with a slave dressed in matching pink attending the guests.[92] Another caliph ordered a feast in yellow. He sat in a golden domed room covered with tapestry of golden brocade, and was served melons, oranges, and yellow wine in golden vessels by slaves dressed in yellow brocade. The water in the fountain beneath the dome was colored with saffron.[93]

The alternation of night and day, a theme mentioned a number of times in the Koran, was another inspiring subject. Ancient Arabic has a multitude of names for every phase of the night. Le Goff writes that "the night was the time of supernatural dangers" for the medieval European man; in the Arab world the night was the time for entertainment and pleasures. Already the idea of the *Thousand and One Nights*, which is of Iranian origin, suggests the notion of the night as the time for leisure and diversion. All forms of Arabic literature associate the night with pleasure. The night is identified with the moon, which is the symbol of human beauty; to be like the moon is the highest praise one can use to qualify a person's looks. The moon signals the Muslim calendar and the time of fasting. Most particularly the nights of Ramadan, between fast-breaking and dawn supposedly spent in prayer, were often devoted to parties and other distractions, story-telling, chanting, and literary recitation. The Koran, moreover, describes the night as the time when truth is revealed: "It is in the watches of the night that impressions are strongest and words most eloquent." (73:6)

Night is the time for artificial light, and has inspired the creation of intricate devices for producing illumination. The candle and the lantern occur frequently in bacchic poetry as symbols of the lover's dreams.

As in the European Middle Ages, gems and precious metals were valued as symbols of beauty. Following ancient traditions the palaces of the Abbasid and Fatimid caliphs had pavilions and gates named for precious stones and metals, such as the hall of gold or the emerald hall. In the *Arabian Nights*, precious stones illuminate an entire hall or palace and radiate a light that brightens the night.[94] Precious stones were also associated with the sea; in the tale of the sea ʿAbd Allāh and the land ʿAbd

Allāh a water creature carries precious stones from the sea, where they were as common as pebbles on land. This may have been inspired by the Koranic text referring to ornaments made of gems from the sea (16:14, 35:12). Stones and minerals were also associated with magic and healing powers. Rubies were worn as deterrents against the plague, and turquoise is still used nowadays to repel the evil eye.

In poetry, precious stones were metaphors for all that is cherished and dear, whether natural, artificial, or abstract. Comparisons with precious metals and stones are features in the topoi of Arabic literature. Abū Ḥayyān al-Tawḥīdī (d. ca. 1023) called calligraphy "jewelry fashioned by the hand from the pure gold of the intellect." Poetry too is compared with the jeweler's art, and a multitude of scholarly books have ornate titles with references to gold, pearls, and gems, such as "the meadows of gold," "the spread of gold," "the cast gold," "the unique necklace," "the gems of wisdom," "the precious gem," "the hidden pearls," "the solitary pearl," "the doll's crown," and "the crown of knowledge."

In the interpretation of dreams, almost all precious stones are auspicious signs for prosperity, progeny, and happiness, and therefore jewelry also portends good fortune for women. Pearls symbolize the Koran and the religious sciences.[95]

Fauna

The world of the pre-Islamic Arab poets was crowded with animals; about eighty different types are mentioned in their odes. Extended description of camels, horses, onagers, and animals of prey form an integral part of pre-Islamic poetry. The description of a she-camel by Ṭarafa reveals not only the fascination with animals, but it is also characteristic of a traditional poetic and aesthetic approach, found in love poetry as well, which relishes piece-for-piece descriptions that highlight details of the cherished object:

> Perfectly firm is the flesh of her two thighs—
> they are the gates of a lofty castle, smooth-walled castle—
> and tightly knit are her spine-bones, the ribs like bows,
> her underneck stuck with the well-strung vertebrae,
> fenced about by the twin dens of a wild lote-tree;
> you might say bows were bent under a buttressed spine.
> Widely spaced are her elbows, as if she strode
> carrying the two buckets of a sturdy water-carrier;
> like the bridge of the Byzantine, whose builder swore
> it should be all encased in bricks to be raised up true.
> Reddish the bristles under her chin, very firm her back,
> broad the span of her swift legs, smooth her swinging gait;
> her legs are twined like rope uptwisted; her forearms
> thrust slantwise up to the propped roof of her breast.
> Swiftly she rolls, her cranium huge, her shoulder-blades
> high-hoisted to frame her lofty, raised superstructure. . . .
> Her long neck is very erect when she lifts it up
> calling to mind the rudder of a Tigris-bound vessel.
> Her skull is most like an anvil, the junction of its two halves
> meeting together as it might be on the edge of a file.
> Her cheek is smooth as Syrian parchment, her split lip
> a tanned hide of Yemen, its slit not bent crooked;
> her eyes are a pair of mirrors, sheltering
> in the caves of her brow-bones, the rock of a pool's hollow. . .[96]

Menageries and aviaries belonged to the regalia of Oriental kings both before and after Islam. Exotic animals were acknowledged as valuable gifts to be presented to kings, along with handsome slaves, gems, and artistic objects.

There is a rich literature dealing with animals, as wonders of the world and as examples of wisdom for man to learn from. The Indian book of fables, *Kalīla wa Dimna*, translated into Arabic during the Abbasid period, became one of the most famous and the most frequently illustrated books in Arabic classic culture. Bestiaries were compiled in all periods. The most famous is Jāḥiẓ's book of animals, which belongs to the *adab* genre and consists of seven volumes where animals are described as wonders of God's creation, with great attention given to their behavior and their psychology. Jāḥiẓ is reported to have considered the three most marvelous things of this world the owl, the crane, and a bird called "the master of sadness" (or heron): the owl, because he never appears by day for fear that his beauty, of which he thinks highly, might attract the evil eye; the crane, because it never rests on two legs at once and because it walks softly; the master of sadness because he watches the water while the tide recedes, fearing that it might disappear from the surface of the earth.[97] Jāḥiẓ was also interested in animals because he saw in them aspects of the human character. The human being, as a microcosm of the universe, combines all its attributes.

A long list of animals is recorded in the literature dealing with the interpretation of dreams, as good or bad omens. Arabic literature and fairy tales mention fabulous animals believed to dwell in the seas and the deserts. Fantastic animals and birds are the friends of humankind: they appear as magical transport carrying people across countries and continents. Mythical animals from pre-Islamic cultures, most of all the dragon, have been integrated in the arts of the Arab world. In the *Arabian Nights* many stories describe metamorphoses of humans into animals. Birds, such as the peacock, the dove, and the crow, often had symbolic associations. The bird was used in esoteric and mystic literature as a symbol of the soul.

The gazelle was a favorite animal for hunting, but it was also cherished for its grace, and remains to this day for the Arab the symbol par excellence of female beauty. The large black eyes of the houris of Paradise are

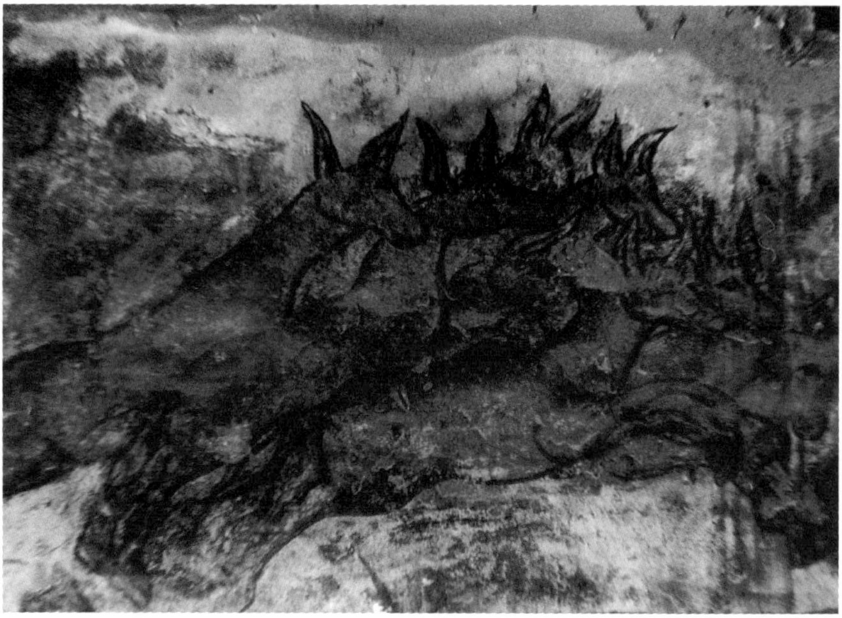

Wall paintings from Umayyad desert palace of Quṣayr ʿAmra, 8th century

compared with those of a gazelle. Even in modern Arabic idiom, comparing a woman with a gazelle attests to her beauty, especially that of her eyes. Many Arabic male and female proper names mean animals such as falcon, lion, panther, and gazelle.

As in many cultures, in literature and in the arts the lion was associated with royal and virile attributes and played a major role in the iconography of kings. It was also represented in heraldic and astrological contexts. Arabic classical literature is said to have more than six hundred words for lion and a similar numbers for camel and horse.[98]

Animal motifs were common in the visual arts. Hares, gazelles, lions, felines, birds and fish as well as mythical animals appear on ceramics, metalware, jewelry, architectural decoration, furniture, and all forms of textiles, even in places such as Mamluk Egypt and Syria, where representations of human figures were scarce. They occur in hunting scenes, which were among the most popular subjects of Islamic art. In the *Arabian Nights* a bride parades "in a robe embroidered in gold with dazzling figures of all kinds of birds and beasts, with eyes and bills of precious stones and feet of rubies and green beryl."[99] Although the Arabs were less interested in miniature painting than the Iranians and Turks, bestiaries and books of fables were often illustrated. The shadow plays included many scenes dealing with real and fabulous animals fighting among each other or being pursued by hunters.

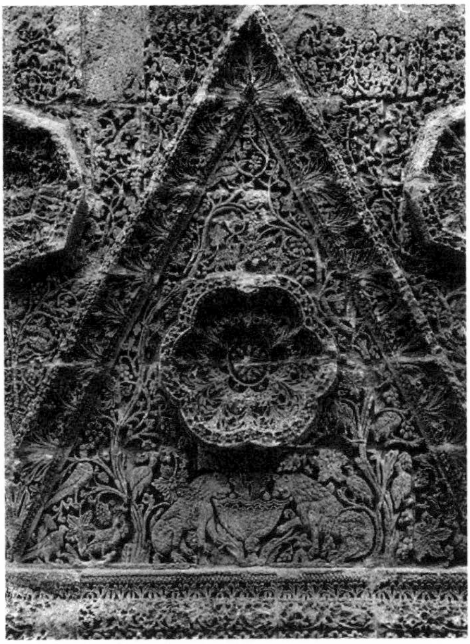

Exterior ornament with lion motif from Umayyad desert palace of Khirbat al-Mafjar, early 8th c. C.E.

Sculpture was not common in Arab culture, but sculptured animals are known, often in association with regal objects. Historians tell about Fatimid caliphs of Egypt having trinkets and sugar sculptures with animal shapes. Lions spitting water were used as bronze aquamaniles and fountain spouts, the most prominent example being at the Alhambra in the Court of the Lions. Following ancient traditions, furniture with feline feet was common.

Unlike humans, animals in Islamic art were depicted dynamically, emphasizing movement; they were usually executed with greater finesse than human figures, which tended to be hieratic. The hunting scenes painted in the 8th century on the walls of the Omayyad desert pavilion Quṣayr ʿAmra emphasize in a spectacular manner the vigor and beauty of running onagers and hounds. But even in 14th-century metalwork, friezes with running animals show their fascination with this theme. Animal forms were also integrated into arabesques where they appear twisted, curled, and entwined.

Human Beauty

Human beauty was a major topic in Arabic aesthetic discourse, and the only subject besides calligraphy for which aesthetic canons were compiled. A special literature deals with female beauty, describing in detail its types, forms, colors, and proportions, and setting criteria for perfection. It also includes a discussion of the tastes and predilections of religious and historic persons for certain women. A large variety of terms were used to describe types of female beauty and grades of beauty and sex appeal. Biographies have been written of slave girls and free women alike who were celebrated for their beauty, intelligence, and culture. Human beauty is treated in all forms of literature in complex terms. According to many theologians, including Ghazālī, God perfected the human image and designed the human being (*ṣawwara*), like an artist (*muṣawwir*) creating an image. *Al-Muṣawwir*, the designer, figures among the traditional names of God. The Koran describes God as having anthropomorphic attributes.

The Koran and religious literature describe how women look in paradise, referring to their eyes, their breasts, their skin, their jewelry, and their clothing.[100] The fascination with human beauty has been most powerfully expressed in the Koran itself, in the story of Potiphar's wife and her love for Joseph:

> In the city, women were saying 'the Prince's wife has sought to seduce her servant. She has conceived a passion for him. It is clear that she has gone astray.' When she heard of their intrigues, she invited them to a banquet prepared at her house. To each she gave a knife, and ordered Joseph to present himself before them. When they saw him, they were amazed at him and cut their hands, exclaiming: God preserve us! This is no mortal, but a gracious angel (12:30–32)

Here, beauty is shown as charismatic and dazzling to the point of disturbing the mind. The friends of Potiphar's wife, who were first contemptuous of her behavior, at the sight of Joseph can no longer blame her, and instead they are themselves captivated by his charm, to the point of losing control over what they are doing, and injuring themselves with their knives. Joseph's stunning beauty is not human, but rather that of a heavenly creature, of an angel. His appearance frightens the women, who pray to God to preserve them.

Beauty confuses the mind and wounds like a knife. It is dangerous. Arab poets compare the gaze of the beloved to a dart that hits and wounds the heart. Ghazālī and Ibn Qayyim compare the gaze to a poisonous arrow and stress its sinful implications, justifying why Islamic law condemns gazing as a sin when it is coupled with desire.[101]

In pre-Islamic poetry the physical beauty of the beloved lady was a major theme. The poet describes the object of his love as well-proportioned like a statue. The whites of her eyes are bright, her face is oval, her nose regular, her neck long, her waist fine, her buttocks strong, her feet well formed.[102] She is of noble descent, fragile, well protected, and generous. There are a multitude of such poetic descriptions, differing little in content, the pre-Islamic pattern having been for centuries copied without much variation.

The following is an excerpt from the ode of Imru 'l-Qays, the greatest pre-Islamic Arab poet (d. 540):[103]

Her slender waist and legs more plump than fine;
A graceful figure, a complexion bright,
A bosom like a mirror in the light;
Her face a pearl where pale contends with rose;
For her, clear water from the untrodden fountain flows.
Now she bends half away: two cheeks appear,
And such an eye as marks the frightened deer
Beside her fawn; and lo, the antelope neck
Not bare of ornament, else without a fleck;
While from her shoulders in profusion fair,
Like clusters on the palm, hangs down her jet-black hair.

For Ibn Qayyim al-Jawziyya, the ideal woman is tall with a slender waist, plump legs, and an ample bosom. She has a fair complexion, long black hair, a long neck, a large forehead, big black eyes with bright whites, black eyebrows; her cheeks are red and her lips pink, her mouth is small and her nose fine.[104]

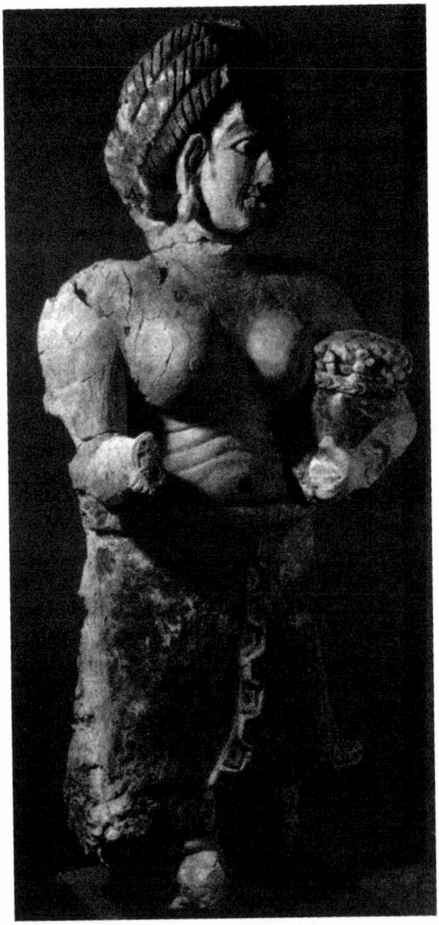

Statue of a woman, Umayyad desert palace of Khirbat al-Mafjar, 8th century.

Ibn Qayyim composed a long lascivious poem which preaches virtue and piety to the Muslims, inciting them to earn the heavenly enjoyment of houris in paradise. In this poem he praises *in extenso* the carnal attributes of the houris, describing every inch of the female body, the charm of its movements, its sex appeal, and its ravishing effect on the senses of sight, smell, and touch.[105]

The hair of the beloved woman is celebrated at length by Arab poets as a major seductive feature; for this same reason it is the subject of detailed regulations in the *Sharīʿa*, which prohibits the Muslim woman to show her hair and allows the man to dye his with henna. The ideal female hair is black, thick, fragrant, falling in waves and sometimes also with curls.[106] The hair is so important in Arab culture that the *Encyclopaedia of Islam* has assigned three authors to write about it, and includes a long contribution dealing with the graying of the hair (*shayb*). In Arabic poetry white hair had gloomy associations, being almost a symbol of evil. In contrast to youth, it epitomized sexual abstinence, decrepitude, solitude, and despair. The poets lament over and over that white hair provokes the disgust of beautiful women. While some wrote ironical apologies of the aged man, many composed poems where the white-haired lover is being ridiculed by women. "The majority of poets seem to imply

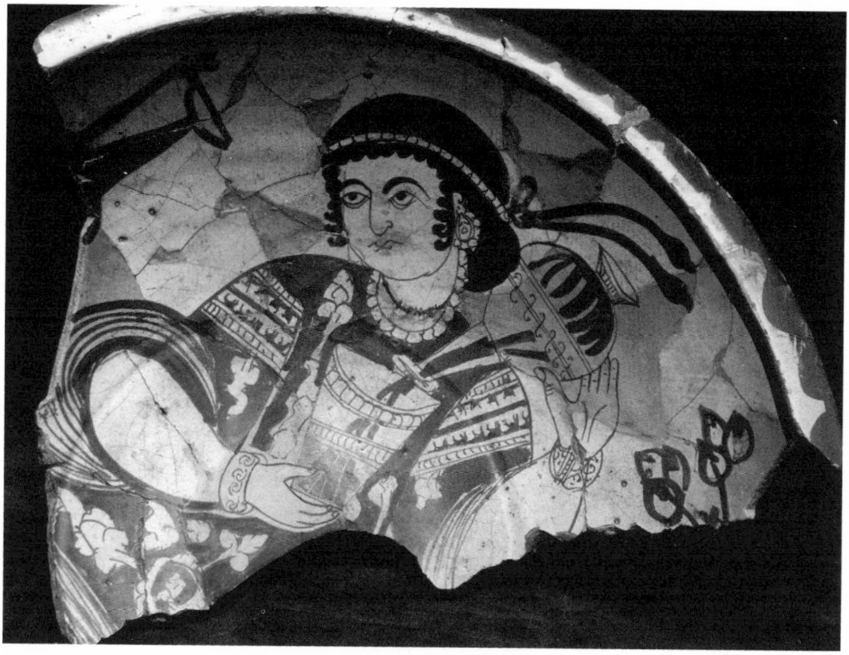

Fatimid plate, Cairo, 11th c.

that the lady has the right on her side."[107]

In spite of their conventional character, the criteria of female beauty were not static. The appearance of a Central Asian, Mongol, and Turkish ruling aristocracy in the Muslim world stimulated an erotic preference for Asian types. This appears in the figural motifs in the visual arts as well as in Mamluk love poetry, where the Turkish type supersedes the Arab as the female ideal.

In bacchic poetry the cup-bearer, who is either a slender youth with curling forelocks or a gazelle-like girl, is as important as the wine itself. The praise of the cup-bearer's looks characterizes this poetic genre. In the *Arabian Nights*, beauty, in whichever gender, is a decisive factor in igniting love. All love episodes begin with an encounter where the beloved is described as having a dazzling appearance. Descriptions of human beauty are idealistic and stereotyped, without much distinction between male and female; beauty is an attribute of both women and men. A lady describes her encounter with a young man in these words:

> There I saw the young man sitting on a high couch, leaning back on a round cushion, with a fan in his hand. A basket was set before him, with fruits, flowers, and scented herbs, as he sat there all alone... so splendidly handsome that he seemed to be cast in beauty's mold. He was like the green bough or the tender young of the roe, ravishing every heart with his loveliness and captivating every mind with his perfection. Faultless in body and face, he surpassed everyone in looks and inner grace.[108]

In another tale, a woman who presents herself as "head of her family, mistress over servants and slaves, and a businesswoman of considerable wealth"[109] depicts the man of her desire in these words:

> When I looked at him, I saw a face as beautiful as the full moon. . . . It was a face on which the supreme God has bestowed the robe of beauty, which was embroidered with the grace of his perfect cheeks.[110]

The face like the moon is an expression used for more than a thousand years and still very current in modern Arabic.

The ideal slave girl in the *Arabian Nights* was "about five feet tall, with a slender waist, heavy hips, swelling breasts, smooth cheeks, and black eyes." She was also knowledgeable in "Arabic grammar and syntax, enunciation and penmanship, jurisprudence and medicine, and the explication of the Quran, as well as the art of playing on every musical instrument."[111] Her price was accordingly high. Many tales involve a hero who spends his entire fortune and all his possessions just to purchase a slave girl he admires. What the tales convey is confirmed by the chronicles, which often mention the astronomical prices paid for the purchase especially of musician slave girls.

In the tale of Ibrāhīm and Jamīla ("the beautiful") a young Egyptian prince falls in love with a woman whose portrait he sees in a book.[112] He abandons everything and sets out for a journey from Cairo to Basra to meet her, enduring all kinds of hardship on his long way. Jamīla lived secluded and well-guarded, refusing to deal with men. Ibrāhīm hides in her garden to watch her. She appears dancing with her female servants, wearing a light shirt embroidered with gold and pearls. Suddenly she spots him and recognizes that he is the man of unequalled beauty whose description she had often heard, and with whom she was already in love, dreaming of meeting him one day and waiting for this moment. Before the happy ending the couple goes through a series of adventures, chased by the painter of Jamīla's portrait who is trying to marry her off to his own son. The subject of this tale is the power of beauty that hits the heart at the first glance, at the sight of a portrait, or even through hearsay.

In love stories the beauty of the one has to be matched by the beauty of the other; both partners are of equal, unheard-of beauty, and each is ravished by the beauty of the other. People come from afar and gather to admire the beauty of a youth; a young man receives sympathy and special treatment, even from his executioner, just because of his good looks. Beauty requires an aesthetic frame, where good fortune and wealth are coupled;[113] the happy ending of a tale brings wealth and glamour, usually in the form of a kingdom, to the handsome couple.

In spite of the established criteria for female beauty observed in poetry and belles-lettres, it was generally admitted that inclination followed individual tastes. Ibn Qayyim writes that, although beauty could be qualified with proportionality, or with the radiance of the face and the eyes, in his view it consisted of a combination of factors. He admitted, moreover, that there were other diverse and individual criteria for determining human beauty.[114]

A story in Iṣbahānī's *Book of Songs* illustrates vividly the perception that beauty was relative and based on psychological criteria. Sukayna, a descendant of the Prophet and granddaughter of the Caliph ʿAlī, had a large abscess near her eye that covered part of her face and had to be surgically removed, which eventually saved her face but left a scar near her eye. This scar was found by everyone to be a most attractive feature, giving the effect of an ornament or jewel.[115]

The relativity of what constitutes human beauty is also illustrated in the description of ʿUlayya, the poetess. She had many talents and great charm, but she also had a physical flaw, an ugly, overly large forehead, which she hid with a special type of diadem. This diadem eventually became a female fashion of her time.[116]

An extreme subjective view of human beauty was expressed by a poet in love who wrote:

> How ugly and unpleasant are people in my eyes if I look and do not see you among them.[117]

The abundance of information about what the Prophet Muḥammad looked like is a rare phenomenon in the history of religions. Descriptions of the Prophet do not represent him as a heavenly creature, but as a human being with no divine attributes, albeit an outstanding man. He is described as being neither tall nor short, not fat, having long curly black hair, very fair skin, dark black eyes with long lashes, broad shoulders, and strong arms and legs. He had a large mouth and beautiful teeth. Even his smile is described in such detail that the Arabist R. Sellheim devoted an article, including a drawing, to reconstructing its exact configuration.[118] Tradition also reports how the Prophet dressed and which colors and perfumes he favored. He loved to perfume himself with musk.

In Arabic historical and biographical literature it was customary to include a description of the subject's appearance. In Mamluk historiography, for example, the character and appearance of the sultans are always included in their obituaries. The portrait was given in plain terms with no attempt to make it conform to the person's character or importance. Great heroes like Ṣalāḥ al-Dīn (1169–1193) and the Mamluk sultan al-Ẓāhir Baybars (1260–1277) were not blessed with impressive looks. Al-Nāṣir Muḥammad (1294–1340), the most powerful in the history of Mamluk sultans, was said to have a limp.

In a society where slaves played an important role, where those purchased to become Muslim soldiers could eventually become sultans and princes, criteria of physical fitness and vigor were of major significance and had to be taken seriously. An entire literature was devoted to the art of buying slaves, to selecting them according to the functions they were required to fulfill. It dealt with criteria for judging the health and character of persons according to their physiognomies and physical features, and it discussed the characteristic features of various races. According to this literature physical features are indicative of character attributes.[119] The concubines and wives of sultans and notables, who became mothers of sultans and princes, were also purchased generation after generation on the slave market, selected according to their physical attributes, especially their beauty. It should be recalled that concubinage with a slave girl was legal in Islam and the children of slave women were legitimate; their legal status was the same as that of children born in marriage. There was no limitation on the number of concubines as there was for the number of wives. The slave girl, unlike the free woman, was not veiled. In contrast to Europe, where ladies of the aristocracy were married for their lineage and dowry, in Muslim aristocratic circles aesthetic criteria usually prevailed in the choice of wives, though political marriages were also concluded. Legal documents dealing with the purchase or inheritance of a slave included a description of his or her physical features.

Biographies of poets and musicians in the *Book of Songs* describe the artists not only in terms of their art and level of performance, but also in terms of their looks, their allure, the elegance of their manners and appearance, their wit, and their impact upon the audience. An artist who combined many talents including spirit, erudition, elegance, and a pleasant character was particularly valued. Refinement was a prerequisite of a singer's or musician's profession; unattractiveness could hinder a musical career. Singers were supposed to show a pleasing physiognomy during their performances; their expression was observed, even studied and copied by others. Al-Gharīd had many talents, but he still "worked at his personality to make himself brilliant" (*kāna yaṣnaʿu nafsahu wa yubarriquhā*).[120]

Many historical personalities in Islam had nicknames referring to their looks, like al-Jāḥiẓ, for example, whose name refers to his protruding eyes. In the *Arabian Nights*, physical faults, such as being one-eyed or hunchbacked, often portend calamity for the character possessing them. In the deed of a pious foundation (*waqf*) it was often stipulated that the attendant of a public water-house, who serves water to the passer-by, should have an impeccable appearance; sometimes it was even required that he should be good-looking. Similarly, the *ḥammām* attendant was expected to have good looks and a nice voice.

According to one *ḥadīth* a good-looking believer is the utmost perfection and an ugly unbeliever is the utmost ugliness.[121] Here, physical beauty is valued as analogous to virtue. Accordingly, one must assume that the ugly believer is less agreeable to God than the good-looking one, and the handsome unbeliever less evil in God's eyes than the ugly one!

Ghazālī describes physical beauty as a blessing (*niʿma)* and power (*qudra*); a good-looking person is more apt to reach his or her goal than an ugly one, as physical beauty is likely to be the reflection of goodness.[122] For this reason beauty was viewed as a useful attribute. Inner beauty manifests itself according to the principle that the face and the eyes are the mirrors of the soul. The Prophet and the saints were therefore believed to have been beautiful.[123] Ibn Qayyim reports that some women preferred to perform their prayer at night because night prayer enhanced the beauty of the face![124] Not all writers, however, identified beauty with goodness; according to some, a good-*looking* person was not necessarily a *good* person; physical beauty could be a lure. As Abū Ḥayyān al-Tawḥīdī said, all that is good is also beautiful, but not all that is beautiful is good.[125]

Some *ḥadīth* texts go very far in emphasizing the value of physical beauty: for example, the one saying that beautiful people are auspicious (*uṭlubū al-khayra ʿinda ḥisān al-wujūh*), or the one that says looking at a beautiful face is a form of devotion (*al-naẓar ilā 'l-wajh al-malīḥ ʿibāda*)[126] are two examples. Another states that water, greenery, and a beautiful face exalt the soul. Such *ḥadīth*s are not universally acknowledged, and they even provoked controversies because they invited unorthodox interpretations, such as the sufi conception that human beauty is a manifestation of God and the love of physical beauty, i.e., erotic love, is a form of venerating God's creation. The identification of the good with the beautiful in human beings was also expressed in poetry, especially in panegyrics.[127] In Arab popular belief today, a beautiful face is still considered auspicious, and an ugly person is believed to bring bad luck.

In the eyes of Ibn Ḥazm (d. 1064), female, unlike male, beauty is fragile and needs care. To illustrate the point he describes an encounter with a beloved lady after a long separation:

> Her charms were greatly changed. Gone was her radiant beauty, vanished her wondrous loveliness; faded now was that lustrous complexion which once gleamed like a polished sword or an Indian mirror; withered was the bloom in which the eye once gazed transfixed seeking avidly to feast upon its dazzling splendor only to turn away bewildered. Only a fragment of the whole remained, to tell the tale and testify to what the complete picture had been. All this had come to pass because she took too little care of herself, and had lacked the guardian hand which had nourished her during the days of our prosperity, when our shadow was long in the land; as also because she had been obliged to besmirch herself in those inevitable excursions to which her circumstances had driven her, and from which she had former-

ly been sheltered and exempted.

For women are as aromatic herbs, which if not well tended soon lose their fragrance; they are as edifices which, if not constantly cared for, quickly fall into ruin. Therefore it has been said that manly beauty is the truer, the more solidly established, and of higher excellence, since it can endure, and that without shelter, onslaughts the merest fraction of which would transform the loveliness of a woman's face beyond recognition: such enemies as the burning heat of the noonday, the scorching wind of the desert, every air of heaven, and all the changing moods of the season.[128]

Women occupy a prominent place in the figural representations found in the visual arts. They are usually depicted in a hedonist context, as musicians and dancers, and in Omayyad art they appear in provocative attire and poses, or half-naked. The half-naked figures in the paintings and sculptures of Quṣayr ʿAmra and Khirbat al-Mafjar were produced in the 8th century at a time when such exuberance was not common in Western art. Khumārawayh, the son of Ibn Ṭūlūn and ruler of Egypt in the 9th century, owned life-size statues of his female singers, adorned with their jewelry.

Al-Jāḥiẓ writes that the pleasure produced by a slave girl who has been selected as a beautiful female musician and singer is due to the fact that she addresses three senses; sight, hearing, and touch. Slave girls thus represent the ultimate seduction. Referring to the *ḥadīth* that warns the believer to avoid the sinful glance of desire, Jāḥiẓ asks desperately how one should then deal with this problem when glance is reinforced by music and dalliance. He also notes that human beauty is not a matter of sight alone, but can be perceived in many ways; formal criteria are only some of them. According to Ibn Khaldūn, man's affinity to the beauty of the human body is fundamental and rooted in his nature, as is his longing for all beauty that can be perceived by sight or by hearing.[129]

Love

Love was a topic not limited to poetic discourse; philosophers, theologians, mystics, and also physicians all dealt with it, dedicating an entire literary genre to the subject. As late as the 16th century the physician and scholar Dāwūd al-Anṭākī wrote about love in his medical treaties.[130] Masʿūdī mentions a symposium that took place in the 9th century in the palace of the vizier Yaḥyā Ibn Khālid al-Barmakī to discuss the topic of love.[131] It was attended by a group of scholars representing different intellectual orientations, whose statements on the subject had a lasting impact on Arabic literature. They discussed love from the philosophical, mystical, physical-medical, and poetical perspectives. Love was defined as based on the likemindedness of the partners; it can be subtle or total, and it was a major cause of suffering, capable of subjugating, intoxicating, and humiliating the lover to the point of annihilation.

Jāḥiẓ distinguishes three types of love. The first is *ḥubb*, which he defines as love of God, of one's home country or family. Next is *hawā*, or desire, the first step toward passion, which is *ʿishq*. *ʿIshq* refers to love of the other sex which, like a disease, can consume the lover. In the mystic sense it makes one blind and deaf to everything but God. A handsome man might love an ugly woman or vice-versa; what seems to be a misjudgment, however, is a choice made on grounds of harmony between souls and hearts.[132] A distinction is drawn between formal beauty and beauty that generates love; the latter is independent of formal criteria. Love is "blind and deaf," that is, not based on judgment, is a saying attributed to the Prophet; or in its universal, more popular version, "love is blind."

From the philosophical viewpoint, the cause of love is beauty which attracts the soul yearning for perfection. The soul seeks therein the similarity to itself. Human beauty conceals a divine factor like a hidden pearl.[133]

Interestingly, the subject of love was treated by two of the most rigorous, antirationalistic, and literalist theologians of Islam, Ibn Ḥazm and

Ibn Qayyim al-Jawziyya. One might not expect, perhaps, theologians who refuted free speculative thinking and philosophy and advocated instead a strictly literal interpretation of the Koran to deal with such an emotional and lyric subject, but in fact rigorous theologians favored the development of belles-lettres and particularly love poetry. Vadet interprets this phenomenon as consistent with their belief in God's anthropomorphic features, as mentioned in the Koran. As a consequence, they were particularly inclined to celebrate the beauty of the human face and body, since God shaped man in His own image.[134]

Ibn Ḥazm is the author of the "Necklace of the Dove," which describes love in all its moral and psychological implications. It deals with love aroused in dreams, by description, by sight, or after a long relationship; love does not follow but rather dictates criteria, thus transforming the lover's taste and personality. Ibn Ḥazm discussed the role of body language, suffering, jealousy, homosexuality, infidelity, and adultery. For him man has to operate between two opposite instincts, one that seeks the good and is guided by reason, and the other which is directed by appetite. He concludes with a chapter recommending chastity and the love of God. Ibn Ḥazm wrote about women in the most deferential terms, contradicting vehemently the opinion that low instincts prevail in women, and that men are more scrupulous. To him love is a supreme pleasure.

> I have tested all manner of pleasures, and known every variety of joy; and I have found that neither intimacy with princes, nor wealth acquired, nor finding after lacking, nor returning after long absence, nor security after fear and repose in a safe refuge—none of these things so powerfully affects the soul as union with the beloved, especially if it come after long denial and continual banishment. For then the flame of passion waxes exceeding hot, and the furnace of yearning blazes up, while the heat of expectation cools down. The fresh springing of herbs after the rains, the glitter of flowers when the night clouds have rolled away in the hushed hour between dawn and sunrise, the splashing of waters as they run through the stalks of golden blossoms, the exquisite beauty of white castles encompassed by verdant meadows—not lovelier is any of these than union with the well-beloved, whose character is virtuous, and laudable her disposition, whose attributes are evenly matched in perfect beauty. Truly that is a miracle of wonder surpassing the tongues of the eloquent, and far beyond the range of the most cunning speech to describe; the mind reels before it, and the intellect stands abashed.[135]

Ibn Qayyim was under the influence of the Barmakī symposium when he wrote his book on the various aspects of love. It is an anthology of poetry, *ḥadīths*, and philosophical texts that discuss the grip of passion, the role of will, bondage, and suffering, and also the illicit aspects of love such as pederasty. Love is more intoxicating than wine, gaze being the cup in which it is served. It is like a spell. The highest rapture is reached when love is accompanied by music and wine; then delight would fill the body, the mind, and the soul; wine being intoxicating to the body, love to the mind, and music to the soul.[136] The perfect pleasure is the one that combines soul and body and includes the pleasures of all the senses, sight, smell, and touch.[137] The lover should enjoy God's mercy and be grateful to Him. Like Ibn Sīnā centuries earlier, Ibn Qayyim declared the love of God to be the most exalted form of love because it purifies the soul. Love beautifies the lover, physically and spiritually.[138]

ʿIshq is passion and metaphysical love; it is an irresistible desire to reach the loved object and thus to attain perfection. It is the aspiration toward beauty which God has manifested in the world when He created man in his likeness. Most Arab authors, including al-Ghazālī, distinguished three levels of love—the natural, the intellectual, and the divine. In philosophy and theology love became equivalent to the search for the eternal and divine truth, and in sufism it referred to the love of God.

Arab poetry glorified all forms of love, the erotic as well as the platonic. Some scholars attribute the courtly love celebrated by the troubadours in the West to Arab origins, inspired either by poetry or perhaps by Arabic philosophy. Despite the legal discrimination against women, when it came to love, women were venerated even to the extent of symbolizing God, as in sufi poetry.

Majnūn ("the Mad") is a famous legendary figure of Arabic poetry and folklore who represents the absolute madness of love.[139] Majnūn, the love-poet mad with love for Laylā, is one of the most celebrated themes of Arabic and also Iranian poetry. His love for Laylā was love for its own sake, regardles of the beloved's qualities. Craving to achieve union with Laylā, Majnūn was tormented and in a bewitched state, loses his judgment and becomes indifferent to life. He ends up leaving society and wandering in the desert among the wild animals, where everything around him revives the memory of Laylā. His love for Laylā is a kind of adoration similar to the one reserved for God. This form of love poetry that epitomized absolute love was adopted by sufis, especially in Persia as an expression of their love of God, which sacrifices everything in quest of the union with Him.

Ibn ʿArabī said about Majnūn's love:

> There are some who in their active imagination contemplate the image of the real being in whom their Beloved is manifested; they thus contemplate His real existence with their own eyes, and this is union with the Beloved in the active imagination; then, in contemplating Him in a union whose delicacy and sweetness surpass any material, concrete and objective union. It is this (imaginative union) that absorbed the spirit of Qays al-Majnūn, who turned away from his beloved Laylā, saying "Go away from me"... because Laylā who was present in his active imagination was more suave and real than the real, physical Laylā.[140]

Arabic culture in general adopted the Aristotelian conception that the body is a major factor in the attainment of human happiness, soul and body being complementary, rather than the Platonic and Christian view, which stresses the autonomy of the soul and considers the body a prison and an obstacle to the soul's liberation. Al-Rāzī (d. 925) refutes the idea that Socrates was an ascetic and claims instead that the Greek philosopher, in the later part of his life, led a normal worldly life.[141] For al-Rāzī "all lawful things are to be enjoyed," as long as they do not imply inflicting injustice or committing murder, "though the advantage lies with those who lean towards the lower rather than the upper limit." Al-Rāzī adds: "But to surpass the lower limit is to quit philosophy and to fall into those Indian and Manichaean and monkish ascetic practices which we have mentioned; it is to abandon the just life and to anger God Himself, by paining the spirit to no purpose."[142]

Unlike Christianity, Islam did not favor celibacy as a form of religious devotion. Ghazālī, who opened the way for the integration of sufism with orthodox thought and who emphasized the inward aspect of religion and the spiritual approach to God's beauty, favored marriage and sexual fulfillment as healthy and necessary to individual as well as social health. It allows man to produce progeny and to achieve the physical equilibrium that is necessary for spiritual and religious life. In his book about Islamic medicine, Ibn Qayyim al-Jawziyya includes a chapter on the merits of sexual intercourse that recalls some modern guidebooks on sexual behavior. He enumerates the advantages of lawful sex as follows: it serves progeny and thus mankind, it stimulates the physical functions of the body and strengthens the nerves. It gives pleasure, which is what paradise is about, with the difference that man in paradise enjoys the pleasure without the requirement of progeny. Finally, sex is necessary to keep the mind off sin. In Ibn Qayyim's view everything that contributes to the consummation of marriage is legitimate, even the playing of music during wedding ceremonies, because God wants people to marry.[143] Ibn Qayyim cites a *ḥadīth* of the Prophet which says, "The world is pleasure and the highest pleasure is a fine woman."[144] The Prophet is reported to have described the ideal woman as good-looking, obedient, and loyal.[145] There are also *ḥadīth*s recommending men to take good care of the sexual satisfaction of their female partners with all the necessary foreplay preceding intercourse. Some historians even record how the Prophet kissed his wife ʿĀʾisha.[146] The acceptance of sexuality as a healthy aspect of life is a decisive cultural difference between Arabic and Western religious thinking, also reflected in their different versions of paradise.

Music and Belles Lettres

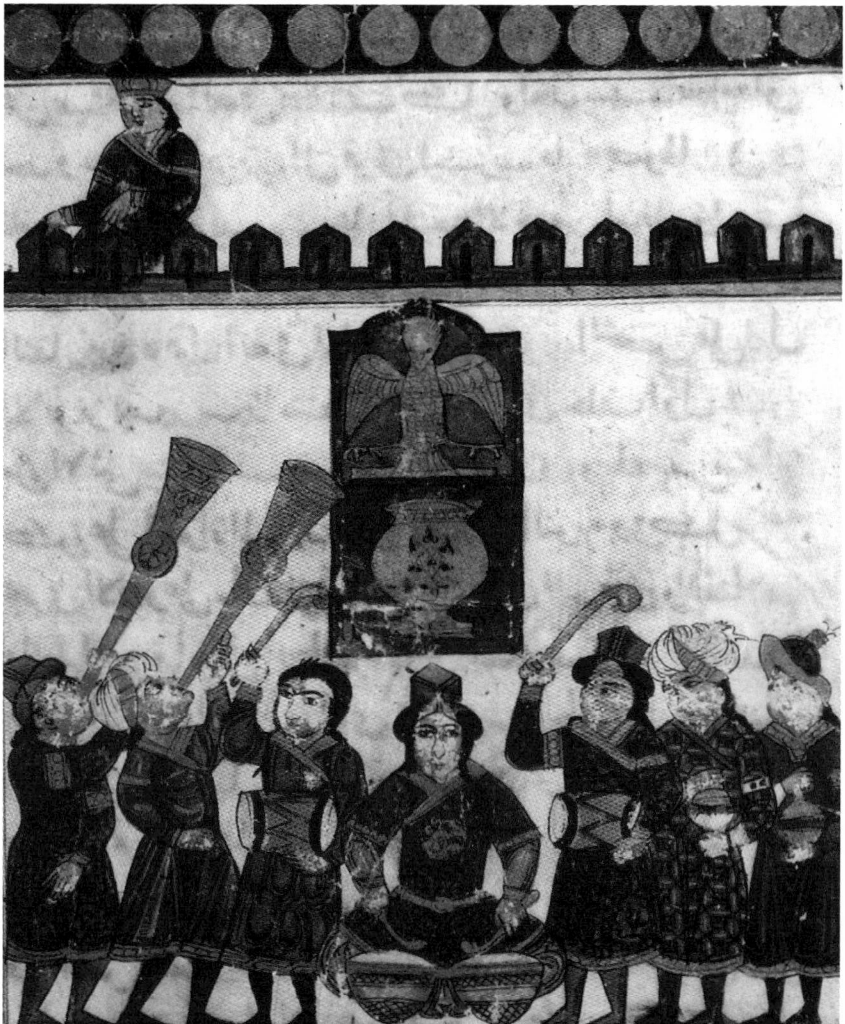

Illustration from al-Jazari's treatise on automata, 13th century.

Music

Music was not only art, it was also science, pleasure, and therapy, a "prescription for physicians to administer to the mind or body of the diseased."[147] Masʿūdī (d. 956) considered the study of music to be the noblest bequest of Greek culture because music ignites and transports the soul; it is the highest of all pleasures and it cannot be grasped by logic. Like many other authors, he believed that there was a correspondence between the human body and the universe and that the humors of the body were tuned to the vibration of music.[148] Farābī wrote that rhythm contributed to nature's beauty; one of his disciples added that the human body itself was rhythmical.[149] The Ikhwān al-Ṣafā distinguished between two aspects of the art of music—the art itself and its psychological effect on people.[150] They adopted the Pythagorean idea that music was an echo of cosmic music produced by the movement of the celestial bodies; it thus reflected the harmony of the universe. Music could produce a perfect emotion which can exalt the soul and repel ugliness. It was to the soul what wine was to the body, pleasure being their offspring.[151] Music could also influence and move animals.

In Arab "mirrors of princes" the authors refer to the sages of Greece, India, and Persia, who described music as both a serious subject and a useful pleasure that educated and cultivated the mind, improved the character, and revived the spirit; that is why it was used by Christians and others in their religious ceremonies. It is therapy for melancholy, and it soothes and inspires children. Music is essential to the well-being of monarchs because of its recreative and healing powers.[152] Scenes showing musicians performing occupy a prominent place in Islamic figural representations. Along with hunting, music was a favorite courtly pastime, depicted on mural paintings and portable objects alike.

The belief in the therapeutic effects of music, or the influence of musical modes on the mind, was based on the Greek doctrine according to which the elements and humors are in relation to particular notes and rhythms, reflecting cosmic order. The philosopher al-Kindī (d. 866), who was also the author of several books on music, was one of the great protagonists of this doctrine; he analyzed the soothing combination of music, colors, and perfumes, a combination which recalls the voluptuous descriptions of courtly pastimes in historical sources and in the *Arabian Nights:*

> And when the arrangement of the rhythms is used in accordance with the periods (of the day) which we have reiterated, along with the employment of the (appropriate) colors and perfumes, according to the disposition of the arrangement which we have mentioned already, the faculties of the soul and its joys appear double of that which appears when employing these things upon the other and individual arrangement which we have described.[153]

The words *ṭarab* and *muṭrib*, which designate music and musician, originally meant "delight" and "delighter." The delight involved here encompasses a wide range of categories, varying from sensual pleasure to the most exalted ecstasy.[154] Ibn Khaldūn regarded music as the most sophisticated form of art because it could only subsist in a highly civilized and urbanized society as an expression of leisure and luxury, devoid of any function other than that of pastime and enjoyment (*kamāliyya min ghayri waẓīfa min al-waẓā'if illā waẓīfat al-farāgh wa'l-faraḥ*). This art is therefore precarious and perishes when its cultural environment declines.[155]

Whereas poetry was conceived to incite imagination and arouse emotion and the visual arts were believed to soothe the spirit and relieve the mood, music was the art to which Arabic literature attributed the most profound impact on the soul. Because of its stirring power which stimulates contemplative activity and leads to ecstasy or intoxication, music can be a profound religious experience or a temptation to promiscuity. For the musician and musicologist al-Kātib (10th/11th century), the true enjoyment of music is not that of immediate emotion, which is the easy access to music, but rather that perceived by a combination of the faculty of audition with that of judgment, and this needs cultivation.[156]

Musical performances at the Omayyad and Abbasid courts were often accompanied by scenes of ecstasy; caliphs are reported to have wept, shouted, fallen on the floor, or torn their clothes in their euphoria. Because of its intoxicating effect, music was celebrated in bacchic poetry. As it was preferably enjoyed together with wine, it came to be identified with bacchic pleasures and hedonism, with taverns and sexuality.[157] According to an old Arabic saying, "The song is the talisman of adultery."[158] For that reason some rulers, following orthodox opinion, prohibited musical performances or allowed them only on a very limited scale. In practice, however, such measures were not very effective, and they remained the exception rather than the rule. Imām Shāfiʿī condemned music as well as everything that is "played," but most of all any music performed by slave girls. Ghazālī quoted Imām Shāfiʿī's and Abū Ḥanīfa's hostile judgments on music, but then argued that there is no statement in the Koran or in Prophet's traditions to confirm such a prohibition. He concludes that since music satisfies one of the five senses which were created by God to provide corresponding pleasures, it cannot be bad. Ghazālī's opinion was endorsed by other theologians, especially among the sufis who, referring to the biblical David tradition and to a *ḥadīth*, considered music an attribute of paradise.[159] In sufi rituals, musical performances, including singing and dancing, were practiced by almost all orders, but the debate over its permissibility virtually never stopped.

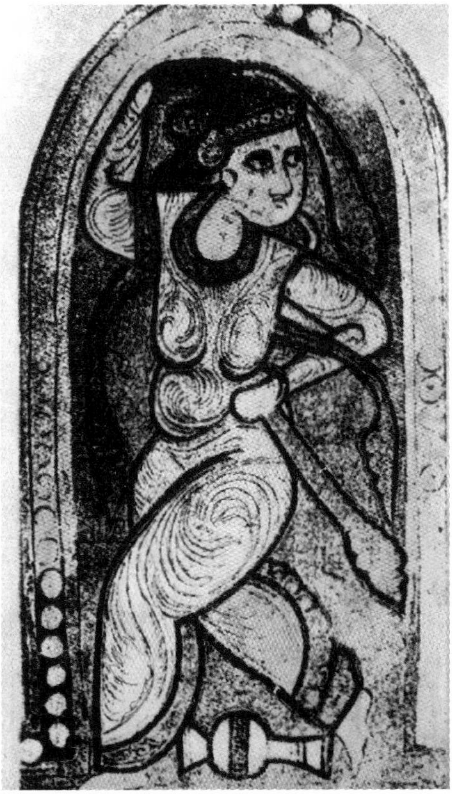
Scarf dancer, detail of painting in the ceiling of the Capella Palatina, Palermo, 12th century.

Advocates of music and poetry such as Ghazālī argued that music, like poetry or language, cannot be sinful *per se*; the moral value of these arts depends rather on their context and use.[160] Music does not generate new feelings in the heart; it only moves those already existing. In a spiritual context it can purify the heart, but associated with evil it becomes illicit. This judgment recognized the mind's freedom and responsibility and viewed music only as a vehicle which, like language, can have various meanings. The senses and the mind are the ultimate critics capable of distinguishing between good and bad. To avoid sinful associations in the listener's mind, however, Ghazālī condemned the use of those musical instruments that were used in licentious performances.

Ghazālī also approved of love songs because they arouse desire, strengthen feelings, and excite pleasure, all of which were permissible on the condition that the relationship between the lovers was lawful. Since concubinage with slaves is legal in Islam, there was considerable room for permissible erotic pleasure. Music, singing, and dance as performed by the Africans were, according to Ghazālī, legitimate because the Prophet had already authorized them as a natural expression of pleasure. Such performances should be allowed on festive occasions and celebrations, for joviality is laudable (*al-surūr mamdūḥ*). He went on even to criticize the antagonists of music as being phlegmatic and incapable of perceiving the beauty of God's creation.

One of Ghazālī's arguments in favor of music was that it is perceived by one of our five senses, which, together with the mind, were created for the purpose of perception. As examples he mentions the musical performances of the Patriarch David and the singing of birds which flatters the ear. He quotes a *ḥadīth* saying that all prophets sent by God had a beautiful voice (*mā baʿatha allāhu nabiyyan illā ḥasan al-ṣawṭ*); a preacher should, therefore, have an elegant harmonic speech to move his listeners.

The Koran is recited in melodic chant and is enjoyed for its musicality; the voice and style of the Koran reciters are praised and discussed in the Muslim world to this day. Many famous singers began their career as Koran reciters. The term *ṭarab* was also used in literature dealing with Koran recitation and with the call to prayer (*ādhān*).

Ghazālī divided the influence of music into two categories, a spiritual and a physical. *Samāʿ* leads the sufi to ecstasy, thus uncovering hidden emotions and purifying the heart; it is an encounter with God. Of this the mystic Dhū 'l-Nūn wrote: "Listening to music is a divine influence which stirs the heart to seek Allāh and those who listen to it spiritually to attain Allāh, and those who listen to it sensually to fall into heresy."[161] Another sufi, al-Darrāj, said, "Listening to music... causes me to find the existence of the Truth behind the veil."[162]

The belief that the fascination with music lies in its power to open up the soul and disclose hidden and secret emotions, revealing them in melodious form, was shared by many thinkers.[163] The essayist and man of letters Abū Ḥayyān al-Tawḥīdī (d. ca. 1023) refers to Socrates as having said that music moves the soul, bringing it back to its sources by freeing it from the alienation of worldly occupations.[164] He adds that the musician, with his art produced by his intellect (*al-nafs al-nāṭiqa*), contributes to the perfection of nature.[165]

In music theory the Arabs both elaborated on and added to the works of the Greeks. Farābī, like his predecessor al-Kindī, was not only a philosopher but also a great theorist of Arabic music; he linked theory with practice and he himself excelled in both. He wrote extensively about improvised rhythmic and melodic ornaments to achieve a higher aesthetic musical effect.

In the Abbasid period musical debates were held at court with the caliph as arbiter. There were different schools of music theory and, as in poetry, the dispute between modernists and traditionalists was a major theme. Isḥāq al-Mawṣilī (d. 850) and his father Ibrāhīm al-Mawṣilī (d. 804) were the most famous musicians of the Abbasid period.[166] Like his father, Isḥāq was the author of an anthology of songs and also collected material about musicians and their craft. He advocated conservative and faithful performances that would not alter the classical music repertoire. His conservative attitude was justified by the fact that music was not written down, so that performance was the only vehicle through which it could be passed on. The conservatives complained that if one followed the practices of the modernists, the musical heritage would have no chance of survival, and it would be lost within a few generations. Isḥāq and his orthodox followers interpreted the modernistic approach as the result of mediocrity, laziness, and the inability to deal with the classical heritage. The modernists, on their side, defended the performer's freedom to impress his personal interpretation on a work, adapting the traditional repertoire to modern taste and requirements. Iṣbahānī admitted that inno-

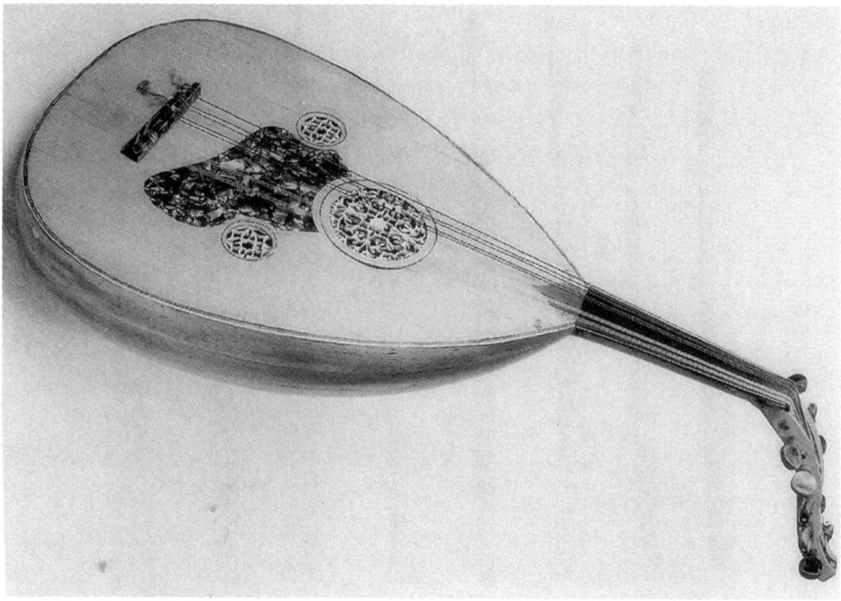

ʿŪd (fretless, short-necked lute)
Musikwissenschaftliches Seminar Göttingen, Inv. Nr. 1262.

vations and fashions were dictated by human behavior: "The human character likes change from one state to the other; it needs novelty to rest from the customary. Novelty is more attractive than custom, and expectation captures the heart more than the present."[167] The debate between modernists and traditionalists continued into the 11th century, when the musicologist al-Kātib wrote in fervent terms in support of the traditional school.[168]

Courtly music always involved vocal performance, the instrumentalist being also a singer and often a poet, whose talent had to combine theoretical with practical ability. A musician had to be equipped with lung power, to master vocal and instrumental intonation and techniques, to have a large repertoire, and to show stylistic versatility, to be creative and original in improvisation, to be capable of genuine feelings, and to have an attractive physical appearance. Those who had every musical talent except a good voice became music teachers at the court.[169] Isḥāq al-Mawṣilī was talented as a poet and musician, but at first his voice was poor. He worked at improving and cultivating it until eventually it acquired a timbre that was celebrated as unique and inimitable.[170] According to al-Kātib, the musician had to combine talent with education. If his listeners were qualified, his performance would have an edifying and exalting influence on their souls.[171] In the society of the 8th-century Hejaz, high-ranking ladies sponsored literary salons (*majlis*) where the musician was also a socialite with gallant manners who enchanted his female sponsor with love songs. In this refined environment, the poet-musician set the rules of elegance and style. Ever since Ibrāhīm al-Mawṣilī, musicians have also taken responsibility for training the next generation of artists. Music schools developed around both male and female musicians.

The *qayna,* a female slave singer purchased to entertain her master, was an institution already known in pre-Islamic Arabia and well documented for the classical period (i.e., before the 12th century). Some of them even married caliphs and gave birth to caliphs. The *qayna* often also distinguished herself as a poet. Her artistic education, of course, increased her price.[172] Although information about these women in the post-Abbasid period is less abundant, the musician slave continued to enjoy a prominent place in Mamluk court life, sometimes also becoming a sultan's wife.

Ibrāhīm al-Mawṣilī was the hero of legends and the protagonist of several tales in the *Arabian Nights* that refer to demonic or supernatural powers as the source of inspiration for the virtuoso's marvelous melodies. Arabic literature abounds in information about musical styles and techniques, the social context of musical performances, the psychological impact of music on the listener, and the religious attitude to music, but it does not say much about the process of musical creation. For this reason, the tales and legends dealing with Ibrāhīm al-Mawṣilī are of particular interest. In one of them, the musician narrates how one evening, while on his weekly holiday at home among his slaves, he suddenly found an old man in his house. Ibrāhīm, quite annoyed at first, could not resist the old man's charm when he began to converse with him about Arabic music and poetry. Neither could he resist the old man's request for him to sing a song, for which he promised a reward. Ibrāhīm sang his song and was surprised when his visitor dared to suggest singing himself. His surprise was even greater after he heard his visitor's performance, which was so exquisite that the walls and furniture of the house seemed to accompany his music! The visitor asked Ibrāhīm to include this song in his repertoire and teach it to his slaves. Then he disappeared as suddenly as he had come, while all doors of the house were closed. Ibrāhīm understood that his visitor was the devil himself. Next day the singer told the story to the Caliph Hārūn al-Rashīd, who asked him to sing the old man's song. The caliph was fascinated and wished the visitor had also come to him. He gave Ibrāhīm a reward, thus fulfilling the visitor's promise.[173]

The same story is reported by Iṣbahānī in his biography of Ibrāhīm al-Mawṣilī, as having been told by Ibrāhīm himself (was it perhaps a ruse to provoke a reward from the caliph?). Iṣbahānī, however, gives another less demonic version of Ibrāhīm's source of inspiration. When Hārūn al-Rashīd asked him how he composed, he answered "I free my mind from sorrows, I visualize the musical pleasure (*ṭarab*), then the melodic path opens itself to me, I follow it, guided by rhythm, and I return triumphant."[174] This story, unlike the previous one, shows that the artist depends for his artistic creation only on his own powers, and needs no supernatural help. Two different traditions are associated here with the musician. A pre-Islamic one, included in the *Arabian Nights*, which attributed demonic powers to the artist, and a rationalistic one, adopted by Iṣbahānī and representing the mainstream of Arab culture, which did not believe in supernatural artistic creation.

Iṣbahānī's book includes numerous stories illustrating the significance of the musician's imagination and creativity in Arab society in the classical period. Innovators and creators of styles (*madhhab*) were famous and their styles were named after them. Musical performance was expected to be creative and to include improvisations adding aesthetic value and uniqueness to a musical interpretation. Because of the importance of improvisation in musical practice, the performer was no less an innovator than the composer or the poet. Alterations or improvisation were creative acts to beautify the music and intensify the pleasure of the audience; they were the ornament of music and had an aesthetic function. Although the audience favored creative performances, conservative interpretations were also admired for their faithfulness to the original and their respect for tradition.[175]

In spite all how much it has changed, through both natural evolution and Western influence, music is perhaps the only traditional art that has survived to the present. It can be used, therefore, to some extent to exemplify traditional Arabic concepts of aesthetics. The aesthetic values and pleasure that Arabs derive from music are akin to those they value in poetry. On this subject the musicologist L.I. al-Faruqi writes:

> The art of the Arabs is an open-ended art, capable of accepting the addition of further motifs and modules if the artist, whatever his medium, so desires.[176]

> The integral role of decoration in the Arab visual arts is not quite dissimilar to that which it has played in ornamentation in Arab musical art. Just as there are an infinite number of motifs which have been combined to form visual arabesques, the musical motif vocabulary of the improvising Arab instrumentalist or vocalist is virtually limitless. When scalar materials permit, motifs move easily from one mode (*maqām*) to another . . . The motif, whether of the visual arts or of music, is never considered to be the most important ingredient in the work of Arab art. Instead, Arab genius is revealed primarily through the manipulation, the structuring of these motifs, through their combination with like and new elements to produce the visual or aural arabesque.[177]

In the contemporary Arab world the interpreter of music is more famous than the composer, because interpretation is regarded as the most creative aspect of the work. Repetitions in musical performances are never identical; when the famous Egyptian singer Umm Kulthūm (d. 1975) gave her legendary concerts, she was asked by the audience to repeat the same stanza up to nineteen times; every repetition had its own improvised melody, each different from the others. A song of twenty minutes could take more than one hour to perform. The Arab judges a concert according to these variations that go on and on and would probably be unbearable to a European audience; traditional music is always the art most difficult for foreigners to understand and appreciate. Because of the basic role of improvisation in Arab music, some critics deplore the modern use of written notes as being detrimental to its innate creative principles.

The art of Umm Kulthūm was perhaps one of the last examples of traditional Arab aesthetics. Her popularity was so immense that critics blamed the Arab defeats in their confrontations with Israel on the diva's songs, with the argument that the audience that would listen for hours to nostalgic, languishing, and sensual love elegies cannot be able to cope with the challenges of a modern society. Umm Kulthūm's songs, with lyrics by great modern poets, deal with love and grief expressed in universal, abstract, and symbolic terms that could arouse nostalgic reminiscences in any listener. The abstract and symbolic character of the nostalgic feelings she conveyed, could even be interpreted politically, especially in times of tension; certain stanzas dealing with the bondage of love were hailed by the audience as expressions of political opposition.

Belles-Lettres

CONTEXT

In the Omayyad and Abbasid periods, poetry was associated with music. Both arts flourished in court circles; they were enjoyed in the harem along with wine and the company of slave girls. Poets and musicians enjoyed great prestige and were generously sponsored; some had careers as glamorous as the Hollywood stars and opera divas of today. Unlike other artists', the originality of their creations was admired and immortalized in historical annals and biographical encyclopaedias. The court poet was a special institution. The Omayyad and Abbasid caliphs themselves belonged to the circle of poets and literary critics, and some of them were also musicians. The Omayyad caliph al-Walīd Ibn Yazīd (743–44)introduced significant innovations in poetry and the son of an Abbasid caliph, Ibn al-Muʿtazz (d. 908), himself caliph only for a single day, was the author of a major work of literary criticism.

Early Islamic poetry was chanted, as Iṣbahānī's *Book of Songs* demonstrates. Iṣbahānī compiled a gigantic anthology of Arabic poetry from pre-Islamic times to the 10th century. In it the poems, or songs, are accompanied by a social history of poetry and music that is full of anecdotes, some of which turn up again in the *Arabian Nights*. Although it includes references to the early days of Islam, the book does not touch on religious themes, but remains exclusively in the profane court circles of caliphs, poets, musicians, and cultivated slave girls. It describes sessions of highly academic artistic discourse and scenes of entertainment and delight, where humor occupies an important place. The union of poetry and music is reinforced by the aesthetic and hedonistic setting.

Poetry was composed for a variety of occasions and purposes; its themes could be panegyric, satirical, lyrical, erotic, bacchic, mystic; it celebrated warfare, nature, the hunt, religion, even events of daily life. Historical literature is full of poems inserted into a text to comment on the events it relates. In the *Arabian Nights* poems are used as a form of

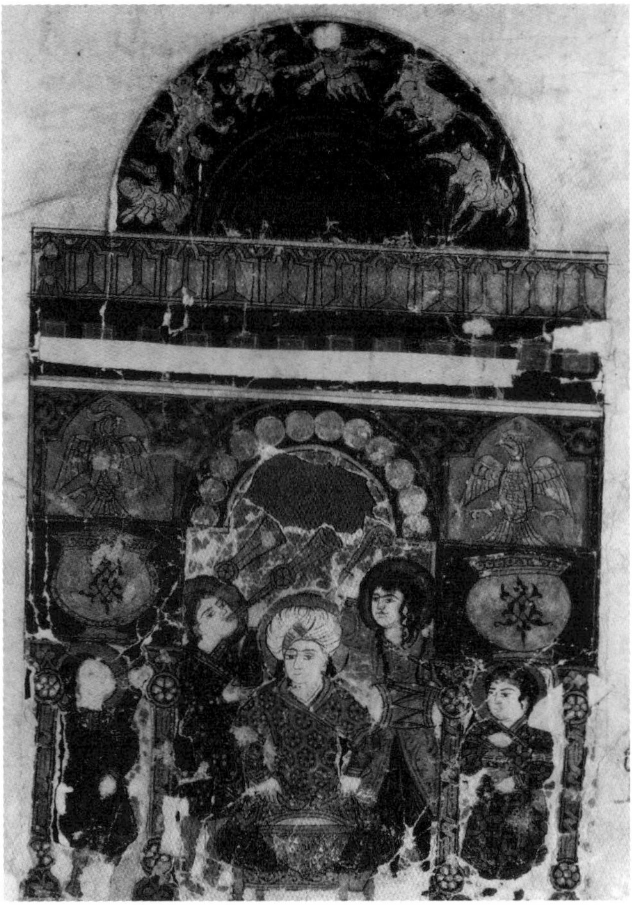

Treatise on automata by al-Jazari, dated 1315.

speech between lovers and as a means of highlighting crucial moments. Poetry was composed not only by professional poets, but also by persons from all classes and both sexes.

Poems were often inscribed on everyday objects such as women's garments, shoes, headgear, handkerchiefs, fans, jewelry, furniture, cushions, curtains, and carpets. They often dealt with love and were used to express the owner's feelings. Iṣbahānī reports that one day the caliph al-Ma'mūn (813–833) read a poem woven on one of his carpets and was so pleased by it that he ordered his court musician, Isḥāq al-Mawṣilī, to set it to music; it eventually became a famous song.[178]

The word *adab* means literature in modern Arabic, but originally it meant a specific type of culture or life-style comparable to the *précieux* culture at the 17th-century French court. The development of *adab* culture in the Abbasid period was an expression of the aesthetic needs of a sophisticated urban society. Vadet describes *adab* as "the social principle par excellence that includes discipline, manners, and ideals through which the individual asserts himself as a member in a group."[179] Originally, the term *adab* meant habit or tradition. With time it came to designate "high quality of soul, good upbringing, urbanity and courtesy." According to Gabrieli it was equivalent to the Latin *urbanitas,* implying urban refinement and culture in contrast to bedouin roughness.[180] It was also used in the sense of etiquette in connection with eating, drinking, dressing, and the art of conversation and erudition. *Adab* as a way of life has been discussed at length in a 9th-century work called *al-Muwashshā* (the embroidered gown); the author who was himself named al-Washshā (the embroiderer), describes in detail what a *ẓarīf*, or gentleman, of the 9th century should be like. He supports his discourse with quotations from the Prophet and other Arab traditions, which we also encounter later in the ethical section of Ghazālī's great book *Iḥyāʾ ʿulūm al-dīn*, indicating that an important aspect of a good Muslim's life is decency in social behavior. The *ẓarīf* is friendly, helpful, thoughtful, sociable, tolerant, and forgiving. He knows how to keep a secret and never resorts to lies. He moves only in cultivated intellectual circles, selecting his friends exclusively from among gentlemen. He speaks little, without haste, and listens the more, as the Prophet recommends. To improve his knowledge, he is not too shy to ask questions. He avoids jokes and buffoonery. He is punctual, tactful, and abstemious. The gifts he makes are small and symbolic such as an apple, a basil twig, or a small perfume flask which the vulgar would disdain. To send a message, the *ẓarīf* write words adorned with silk threads tinted with gold, musk, or saffron. He formulates his text with great care and elegance and inserts poems in his letters. Flowers and fruits belonged to the daily life of a 9th-century Arab gentleman, especially roses and apples, which recall the cheeks of the beloved as they are described in poetry.

An elegant man should never allow himself to become obese; he eats with small bites in moderation. He avoids fat, heavy or smelly foods, as well as beans, garlic, onions, or anything else that produces flatulence. He does not dirty his fingers or mouth while eating, nor does he laugh too much or leave the table before the others.

Al-Washshā dedicates an entire long chapter to the hygiene and aesthetic of the mouth and teeth, often quoting sayings of the Prophet. A favorite gift in the *ẓarīf* milieu was the toothbrush, because of its association with the aesthetic of the mouth and the significance of the mouth in love poetry. Further chapters deal in detail with proper talking, sitting, and walking and with behavior in the streets and markets. The *ẓarīf*'s clothes should be refined and discreet, not showy or in any way resembling female fashion. Only certain perfumes and gems are regarded as appropriate. The female equivalent of the *ẓarīf*, the *ẓarīfa*, or lady, has similar rules for dress. However, Al-Washshā does not limit himself to discussing such refinements. An important section of *al-Muwashshā* is devoted to an anthology of poetry cited on social occasions or inscribed on objects of daily life.

Arab culture honored the gourmet. According to the ideals of *adab* culture, a gentleman should know about the art of cooking, just as he should be informed about equestrian sports or grammar. As a guest, he should be able to quote suitable poems at table and converse about culinary matters. The literary gatherings of the caliphs in the classical period of Baghdad dealt not only with exalted themes of poetry and music, but also with all aspects of life including cuisine. Poets celebrated good food, and a number of medieval authors compiled books on cooking, in which, as in any other literary genre, they quote the Koran, the *ḥadīth*, and philosophical and historical literature. They considered the art of cooking to be a cultural achievement that deserved to be cultivated and documented. The cook was expected to possess specific physical attributes and technical abilities, and his kitchen was supposed to be adequately equipped. The books contain recipes, varying in detail and accuracy, and references to the tastes and preferences of famous persons, often accompanied by anecdotes from a courtly context.

One of these anecdotes is reported by Masʿūdī in his *Meadows of Gold*.[181] It demonstrates how highly Abbasid society valued wit and linguistic finesse and even combined it with religious culture. Abān, a Koran reciter, sat one day together with Hārūn al-Rashīd eating chicken and *harīsa*, a kind of dip, from a dish set between them. The *harīsa* was served with a hollow in its middle filled with chicken fat. Abān, tempted by the fat, did not dare to stretch his hand before the caliph to dip his bread in it. He did, however, make a little depression to let the fat run to his side. Al-Rashīd, noticing this, commented with a verse from the Koran (18:71): "Have you scuttled it in order to drown those on board?" Abān replied in turn with another Koran citation (7:57): "We are pushing it towards a land parched by drought."[182] This playful dialogue at a *harīsa* meal was reported to Masʿūdī by the grammarian Niftawayh, who heard it from Ibn Ḥamdūn, a boon companion of the caliph al-Muktafī, who entertained the caliph at dinner with this anecdote about his famous ancestor.

Some cuisine books were theoretically oriented, more concerned with lexicographical subjects than with recipes, but generally this literature provides abundant information about the culinary traditions of the Arab world. Descriptions of dishes can be also found also in other literary forms. ʿAbd al-Laṭīf al-Baghdādī, the physician who described Egypt in the 12th century, includes descriptions of food in his account. The significance attributed to the art of cooking conforms with the traditional hospitality of the Arab world.[183]

The caliph al-Muʿtaṣim (833–42) organized a culinary competition where each contestant was required to present a dish to be evaluated; al-Maʾmūn was an amateur cook.[184] The caliph al-Muktafī (902–8) was also interested in culinary poetry, and al-Mustakfī (944–46) invited people to a gourmet symposium to discuss poetry dealing with food and cooking. Among the poems presented on this occasion was one on the beauty of asparagus as a plant and as a dish:

> Lances we have, the tips whereof are curled,
> Their bodies like a hawser turned and twirled,
> Yet fair to view, with ne'er a knot to boot.
> Their heads bolt upright from the shoulders shoot,
> And, by the grace of Him Who made us all,
> Firm in the soil they stand, like pillars tall,
> Clothed in soft robes like silk on mantle spread
> That deep hath drunk a blazing flame of red,
> As if they brushed against a scarlet cheek

Whereon an angry palm its wrath doth wreak,
And as a coat-of-mail is interlaced
With kinks of gold so twine they, waist to waist;
Like silken *miṭrāf* that the hands display!—
Ah, could it last for ever and a day!—
They might be bezels set in rings of pearl.
Thereon a most delicious sauce doth swirl
Flowing and ebbing like a swelling sea;
Oil decks them out in cream embroidery
Which, as it floods and flecks them, fold on fold,
Twists latchets as of silver or of gold.
Should pious anchorite see such repast,
In sheer devotion he would break his fast.[185]

Another poem was composed on a pastry called *qaṭā'if*:

When in my friends the pang of hunger grows
I have *qaṭā'if*, like soft folios;
As flows of lambent honey brimming white
So amidst other dainties it is bright,
And, having drunk of almond-essence deep,
With oil it glitters, wherein it doth seep.
Rose-water floats thereon, like flooding sea,
Bubble on bubble swimming fragrantly;
A foliated book laid fold on fold—
Afflicted hearts rejoice when they behold;
But when divided, like the spoils of war,
All have their heart's desire, and sated are.[186]

The following verses celebrate another sweet delicacy:

Its aroma would make even a stone
Open to let it in.
The delicious scent rises
From the place in circles,
The butter drips in spirals.
Its outward appearance
Matches its inner virtue;
Its beauty makes its flavor
Even more exquisite.
The inside is heavy,
But it is enfolded in something

As light and airy
As a spring breeze.
. . . .
Knowing gourmets have rivalled
One another in the severity
Of their criteria for choosing
The kind of sugar used.
Eyes will not tire of gazing
Upon it and the teeth
That sink into it shall never
Be set on edge."[187]

Adab also had bearing on culture and entertaining erudition, including poetry, rhetoric, and Arab tradition. With time its meaning broadened to include a more cosmopolitan form of *humanitas*, embracing Iranian, Indian, and Greek culture. According to Arkoun, "*adab* is literature, poetry, language, history, geography, education, the social code of good behavior, scientific skills that can be mastered in a rational and educated way, and professional activities, especially those of the officials in the administration of the Caliphate."[188] It was the non-religious culture.

The literature of *adab* had Jāḥiẓ and Ibn al-Muqaffaʿ as its most prominent authors. It was light, pleasing, humorous, rational, cosmopolitan and enlightened. It tackled a broad variety of subjects and had to be interesting and not tiring, witty and erudite but not too scholarly. It presented entertaining information to the reader spiced with light comments. In his book *al-Bukhalāʾ*, for example, al-Jāḥiẓ analyzes avarice, in which he portrays human types and social groups such as landlords and pimps. His curiosity encompassed sociological, anthropological, and psychological themes.

Excessive aesthetism and the prevailing elitism of the Abbasid period may explain the growth of an interest in the vernacular and even in the underworldly as a reaction. Literary symposiums were organized to inform the caliphs about the manners and idioms of craftsmen. The taste for the underworld found its expression in another genre whose heroes were eloquent vagabonds and beggars.[189] The famous *Maqāmāt* or "stations" of Ḥarīrī belong to this category.

Unlike the Persians, the Arabs did not regard their myths as belonging to classical literature. They cultivated, instead, history and biography to an extent unparalleled elsewhere in the Muslim world. The 13th-century historian Ibn al-Athīr writes that, unlike prose, a good poem should not exceed a certain length, otherwise its quality would suffer. He notes furthermore that the Arabs were not inclined to produce works like Firdawsi's *Book of Kings*, which is an epic poem as venerated by Iranians as the Koran. The story of Joseph and Zulaykha (Potiphar's wife), which is related in the Koran, was a particular inspiration for Iranian tales and poems, including sufi interpretations of the love theme, but ignored by Arab authors. In Arabic culture the mythical, fabulous, and narrative genres found their outlet in vernacular literature such as the *Arabian Nights* and popular historical romances such as those of ʿAntar and Baybars. In the *Arabian Nights* the tales that have Arab origins are easily recognizable as being less fantastic than those of Persian origin; they often include historic figures and events related in the chronicles, as well as the stories dealing with the urban milieu, the market-place or a merchant's house. Shadow plays, a form of pre-modern theater, were enormously successful in princely as well as in popular circles, but their language was vernacular. Because of their hedonism and pornography, even today the *Arabian Nights* and the shadow plays are a source of controversy and embarrassment, and Arab publishers make ample use of censorship when they publish them.

Bacchic poetry or *khamriyyat* had an acknowledged place in Arabic literature.[190] In between hedonistic and mystic images, it often expressed existential despair. Sufi poets used the *khamriyya* to express the ecstatic and intoxicating love of God. Wine drinking was not the pastime of the solitary, however, but rather a "symposium," a ceremony with its own protocol, whose rules were set in the Abbasid period. It was supposed to be a cultivated, not vulgar, gathering characterized by esprit and art. The *nadīm* (boon companion) was required to have intellectual and aesthetic qualities similar to those of the *ẓarīf*; specialized manuals were written on the etiquette required of him. The aesthetic and erotic features of the cupbearer were extensively celebrated in poems; the setting, which included music, and the objects related to the ceremony of drinking were also of great significance. Poets have composed poems to adorn drinking vessels, and they have praised the beauty of the cup as enthusiastically as they praised its content. For the cup, glass was preferred even to gold.

The brief *khamriyya* poem toasts the luminosity of the wine shining in a glass like a flame, a ray, a star, or a lightning. Wine was called by a multitude of names, according to its color, vintage, and provenance. Its colors were gold, amber, carnelian, or ruby. The wine cup glittered, shedding light into the night like a glass oil lamp; it was compared with a lantern in a prayer niche, thus alluding to the Koran's Light verse, and putting wine in the place of God.

The most famous bacchic poet was Abū Nuwās. He wrote some blasphemous poems, but was not the only great poet to do so. The best Arab poets were known for blasphemy, even heresy. Abū 'l-Ṭayyib al-Mutanabbī (d. 965) (Mutanabbī means "prophecy pretender") was and still is considered one of the greatest Arab poets, if not the greatest. But he dared to pretend he was a prophet and was even reported to have composed a Koran.[191] Similarly, Abū 'l-ʿAlāʾ al-Maʿarrī, another great poet, was openly atheist. He made fun of the Kaʿba and ridiculed the pilgrimage and other tenets of the faith.

> We mortals are composed of two great schools.
> Enlightened knaves or else religious fools.[192]

The Arab poet was by no means a rebel against the norms of society, however. Rather, the poet lived within the liberal rules of a society that respected the profane arts and gave them freedom.

Despite the Prophet's hostility to poets and the rejection of music by puritanical theologians, poetry and music were highly celebrated in Arabic culture. The hostility of the ultra-orthodox could not prevent the practice of these arts, but rather contributed to the progress of their non-religious orientation. The mainstream of poetry and music remained devoid of any linkage with moral or religious values, being rather in conflict with them. Literary criticism continued to consider the pre-Islamic poetic tradition the standard for artistic quality. With their emphasis on formal aesthetic and stylistic criteria, combined with their hedonistic associations, poetry and music remained essentially in the profane domain, and were not expected to fulfill any moral functions.

For the critic Qudāma Ibn Jaʿfar (d. ca. 932), the good poet is the one who masters the art, whatever the subject matter and whether or not it is moral, just as a carpenter's workmanship is not affected by the quality of the wood.[193] Whatever the subject matter may be, good or evil, moral or obscene, the poet's main goal should be literary quality. Sincerity is not the issue—sincerity can be required of prophets, not of poets.[194] Ibn Rushd, commenting on how Arab poets could operate aesthetically even with ugly subjects, such as retreating from battle, said: "You Arabs have made everything look beautiful, even running away."[195] Al-Aṣmaʿī (d. 828) made a radical and famous statement to emphasize the non-committed aesthetic function of poetry, saying that poetry is approached through the gate of sin (*al-shiʿr bābuhu al-sharr*). These words imply that poetic quality is incompatible with morality. Another anonymous poet expanded on this idea, adding that poetry is associated with sin; if it became involved with morality, it would degenerate (*al-shiʿr nakad bābuhu al-sharr, fa idhā dakhala fī 'l-khayr fasada.*)[196] It should be recalled that ravishing musical performances were attributed to the devil (*iblīs*). Some thinkers, however, who adopted the Platonic concepts of beauty, such as al-Rāzī and Miskawayh (d. 1030), disapproved of aesthetic-oriented art and condemned love poetry and romances as frivolous and immoral.[197]

Ibn Sīnā qualified Arabic poetry as mainly aesthetic. He described it as essentially subjective, made to move, please, and impress without being bound by moral or ethical purpose.[198] In these attributes it differed from Greek poetry, which was not composed for mere pleasure but, as narrative or epic, was purposeful and engaged, intended to influence moral conduct.

> The Arabs used to compose poetry for two purposes: (i) to affect the soul by presenting a given matter that moves it in the direction of an action or emotion, and (ii) for pleasure alone—everything was imitated for the pleasure of imitation. On the other hand, the Greeks intended by means of speech, to induce or prevent action. Sometimes they did this by means of oratory, sometimes by means of poetry.[199]

Meter, rhyme, and exalted language provide the framework for the Arabic poem. Rhyme, which was unknown in most early literature, characterized Arabic poetry long before it was generally adopted in Europe.[200] Similes and metaphors were, as Arberry remarked, the bread and butter of the pre-Islamic poet and of his urban successors as well. Western scholars love to apply the term arabesque, when describing Arabic poetry, to refer to its subtle ornamental character and its concise wording. The idea was to create intricate patterns of thought with a minimum of words.[201] Wit and elegance rather than grand meanings were required. As a result, description was often composed for its own sake; startling, almost fantastic similes adorned the poems to the extent of artificiality. Poetry sometimes expressed the poet's virtuosity rather than his sincerity. An anecdote is told about a vizier who during a journey chose to make a stop in a ghastly place called Nūbihār, rather than a more comfortable place, only because it gave him the opportunity to send a letter with a rhymed heading: *Min Nūbihār fī niṣf al-nahār* ("from Nūbihār at midday").[202] Another extreme example of mannerism occurs when poets describe the pyramids of Giza as a pair instead of three for the sake of symmetrical images or in order to compare them with a woman's breasts![203]

An extreme aesthetic view of poetry is the one mentioned in Iṣbahānī's *Book of Songs* or *Kitāb al-Aghānī:* "Not all songs have a meaning and not all that is meaningful has a glamour that pleases the viewer and entertains the listener."[204] Jāḥiẓ and other critics emphasized the aesthetic character of poetry to the extent of rejecting its translation as detrimental to its beauty.[205] For Jāḥiẓ meanings are everywhere; the problem is to give them a seductive and moving formulation. Poetry is a technique or an art (*ṣināʿa*) comparable to painting and weaving.[206] Similarly, for Ibn Sīnā meanings are shared by all, but exalted speech is achieved only with effort.[207]

In writing about medieval European aesthetics and literary criticism, De Bruyne noted that: "The best articulated art theory in the Middle Ages is certainly that dealing with literature."[208] This applies to Arabic culture, as well. The debate on the duality of meaning and expression, or content and form, which was a major topic in Arabic literary criticism, had its roots in the domain of theology and the exegesis of the Koran. Whereas the Muʿtazilites interpreted some passages in the Koran as allegoric, the Ashʿarīs, their antagonists, insisted on a literal interpretation. This became an endless debate on the meaning of image in literary speech that went on for centuries.

In spite of the high value given to skill and technical mastery, virtuosity for its own sake and excessive stylistic embellishments did not escape the criticism of medieval authors. Al-Ḥarīrī (1054–1122), the author of the *Maqāmāt,* was among those who were criticized for their stylistic pirouettes. The *Maqāmāt,* described by Nicholson as "a romance of literary bohemianism," contains a series of detached episodes or sketches dealing with the travels of a cynical vagabond who makes his living by begging or by swindle, using wit and rhetoric for his purposes. The *Maqāmāt* genre is a purely Arabic invention; it was not invented by Ḥarīrī, but it was his book, written in rhymed and rhythmic prose, that became a best-seller at that time. A linguistic *tour de force*, it was compiled essentially to display verbal virtuosity. Its cynical content provoked some protest. In the introduction Ḥarīrī wrote:

> I composed, in spite of hindrances that I suffered
> From dullness of capacity and dimness of intellect,
> And dryness of imagination and distressing anxieties,
> Fifty *Maqāmāt,* which contain serious language and lightsome,
> And combine refinement with dignity of style,
> And brilliancies with jewels of eloquence,

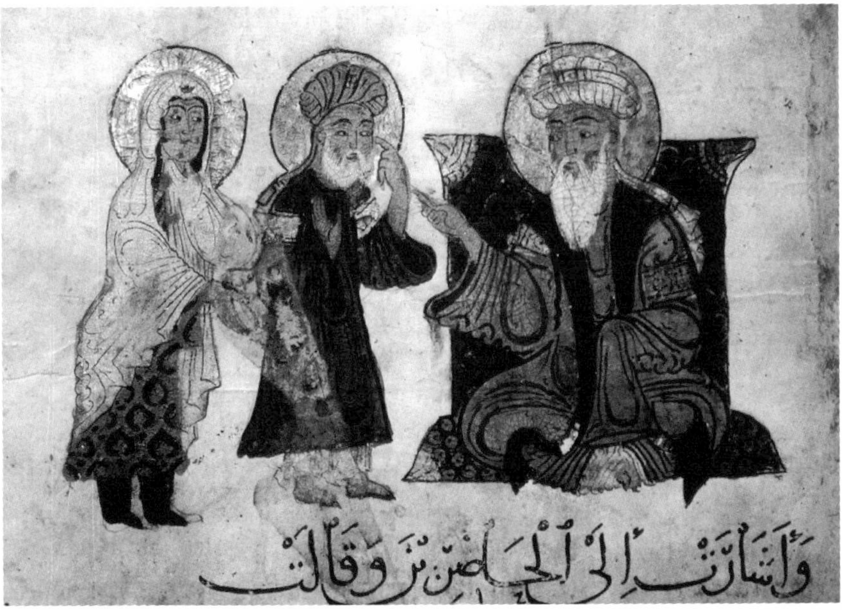

Illustration from "Maqāmāt." Syria or Mesopotamia, prob. 13th century.

And beauties of literature with its rarities,
Beside verses of the Koran wherewith I adorned them,
And choice metaphors, and Arab proverbs that I interspersed,
And literary elegancies and grammatical riddles
And decisions based on the (double) meaning of words,
And original discourses and highly-wrought orations,
And affecting exhortations as well as entertaining jests[209]

The immense success of the *Maqāmāt* is indicative of the aesthetic disposition of medieval Arab society. The hero was an immoral person who made his living using doubtful methods and, as a consequence, was continually in trouble. Thanks to his eloquent poetic pleadings, however, he could reckon on everyone's tolerance and forgiveness. In the end he died as a good Muslim, after having duly repented.

The *Maqāmāt* was the most frequently illustrated book in the medieval Arab world, suggesting that its content was not overshadowed by the preciosity of its style. The reader could enjoy the ambiance conveyed by the narrative and enhanced by the miniatures. The lively and colorful illustrations produced in 13th-century Baghdad and copied in the following century in Cairo depict a variety of scenes from urban life in a style that conveys the jesting and caricatured character of the sketches. According to Grabar the *Maqāmāt* illustrations express the sophisticated taste for art and literature among the Arab urban bourgeoisie between the 12th and 14th centuries.[210] On the literary level, it represented one of the rare forms of fiction that acquired a classical status. Excerpts from the *Maqāmāt* referring to death were even inscribed on a 14th-century prince's mausoleum in Cairo, instead of the usual Koranic verses.[211]

LITERARY CRITICISM

In pre-Islamic Arabia the poet was believed to be inspired by *jinn*s or demons; under the influence of Islam this notion disappeared, and poetry became a profane art. The belief remained, however, that poetry had ravishing and enchanting powers, as did the other arts. Unlike the Greeks, however, who considered poetry a gift rather than a science, the Arabs emphasized the artistic and technical aspects of poetry, which require study and skill. This principle did not exclude the basic belief that God's assistance lay behind any human endeavor. Poetry had to be mastered professionally, like any other craft (*ṣināʿa*),[212] and it had to be practiced with adequate technical tools. A poet works at his theme, endlessly fashioning and remodeling it, like a jeweler operating with precious metals.[213] Technical terms referring to textile, embroidery, or jewelry were regularly used in the vocabulary of literary criticism to describe the poet's work. Masʿūdī, in the epilogue of his great historical encyclopaedia, compares himself to a man who, "having found pearls of every kind and every shade scattered here and there, gathers them into a necklace and makes of them a precious piece of jewelry, an object of great worth which its purchaser will cherish with care."[214] Thaʿālibī, writing about the poetry of al-Mutanabbī, uses terms such as "he moulds the most splendid ornament, and threads the loveliest necklace, and weaves the most exquisite stuff of mingled hues. . . ."[215]

Because poetry was believed to require long training and considerable knowledge (*ʿilm*), experience, and discrimination, some critics, such as the 10th-century author al-Āmidī, went so far as to restrict the competence to judge it to specialists, arguing that an ordinary audience is not able to reach an adequate judgment.[216] ʿAbd al-Qāhir al-Jurjānī expected the audience to be endowed with sharp enough minds to enable them to value good poetry. As for the poet, he should work hard and dive deep to find the pearl.[217]

The emphasis on technical mastery, however, did not entirely exclude the notion of inspiration and talent in Arabic literary criticism. Without talent or inspiration, effort would produce poetry that was awkward, artificial, and stiff.[218] Emotion was also significant: the word *shiʿr* for poetry comes from *shaʿara* which means to feel. However well observed the technical rules, there is a moment when only psychological or emotional criteria can decide what is good poetry and what is not. Poetry articulates deep and hidden feelings and reveals emotions; it was regarded as "white magic." According to Ibn Ṭabāṭabā, harmonious poetry reaches the soul and "it penetrates more powerfully than the spells of magic, more subtly than the sorcerer's charm, more enchantingly than singing;. . . it is like wine in the gentleness of its mysterious spreading, its enchantment, thrill and excitement."[219] Two poems that are equally perfect from the technical viewpoint may have a different emotional impact on the recipients.

According to the poet Abū Tammām (d. ca. 845), "poetry should flow sweetly through our hearts like a stream caressed by basil."[220] The word *dhawq* (taste) and *tadhawwuq* (appreciation) were often used to define the inexplicable psychological predilection for one style over another.

In poetry as in the case of musical performances, there was in the 9th century a debate between modernists and traditionalists, which centered on the notion of spontaneous or natural (*maṭbūʿ*, from *ṭabʿ*, meaning nature) versus artificial poetry. Traditionalism was equated with the natural and modernism with the mannered and artificial. The definition of these qualities remained vague and rather arbitrary; it was often motivated by fear of popular innovations or aimed at disqualifying poets of non-Arab origin.[221]

Fame and success were considered evidence of a poet's quality, because they measured the psychological impact of his work. Since fame could also be due to social and personal circumstances, however, critics agreed that fame had to reach beyond the social circle of the poet before it was a reliable criterion for judging the quality of his work. The controversy over the poetry of al-Mutanabbī is case in point. Some considered him one of the best Arab poets ever; others were equally critical of his work. A whole literature was written to deal with the Mutanabbī case. Advocates stressed his skill and his success as evidence of his quality; opponents accused him of plagiarism and lack of originality. Mutanabbī eventually won the battle, and the consensus remains to the day that his good qualities outweigh his shortcomings. This method of balancing value—measuring the proportion of good against bad qualities—was very common. It was used to make literary assessments of poets and to judge the deeds of monarchs.

Modern critics describe the Arabic poem as being made up of individual elements that can be detached without seriously affecting the whole; as a collection of gems rather than an entity. The Arabs themselves, as Ibn Khaldūn observed, favored poems in which each verse was autonomous, with a complete meaning of its own; it could be detached from the rest and still be significant in itself.[222] The origin of this approach lies in the ideals set by the rhetoricians, whose primary goal was the exegetic analysis of the Koran. They analyzed artistically patterned speech in terms of the basic relationship between word and idea, without dealing with the larger context of a passage. Some poets and critics, however, did not limit their view to this linear perspective and set out to stretch the rhetorical approach to larger units, tackling the issue of the thematic congruence as well. As a result, statements envisaging the aesthetic perspective of the poem as a whole can also be found in Arabic literary criticism.[223]

In his discourse on poetry Ibn Khaldūn confirms the traditional view that poetry is a craft that needs to be learned. He adds that this art has its own complex methodology (*uslūb*) to serve the meaning (*maqṣūd*). Meanings, however, are not the poet's main problem; they exist already in all minds. Meaning is like water, which assumes the shape and color of its container; the poet's role is to form the proper container. Good poets should not overload their verses with meanings.

Ibn Khaldūn considers most religious poetry inferior because of its reliance on commonplaces.[224] In his view, poetic formulations and embellishments are altogether unsuited to expository prose. To master the art, poets have to be familiar with the classical Arabic heritage. They must work within a certain framework, like a weaver at a the loom or the mason on a wall. Mastering the technique does not mean that poets cannot express their own genuine and fresh perceptions. To fulfill this purpose they should not compel themselves to work, but wait for the right mood. Ibn Khaldūn, following older sources, describes poetry as the register of the pre-Islamic Arabs, which summarized their life, wisdom, and history. He ascribed the high quality of classical poetry to the patronage of cultured and refined monarchs who were capable of literary criticism. In later periods, when the monarchs were no longer of Arab stock and no longer fluent in the Arabic language, they were easy to satisfy with mere panegyrics. The quality of patronage and criticism suffered, leading to the decline of poetry.

The first crisis in the evolution of Arabic poetry was prompted by the Crusades and the Mongol invasion, when mourning and nostalgia began to dominate the poet's spirit. Religious poetry became common in Egypt and Syria under the Mamluks, who were generous patrons of religious institutions. With the diminishing interest in poetry, however, the court poet as an institution disappeared and poetry became increasingly a popular rather than a courtly art. Most of the late poets were bureaucrats in the state service. Historians inserted poems in their accounts, commenting on current events, discussing social or political issues, fulfilling a function similar to that of modern editorials. This type of poetry, often written in a casual style, was down-to-earth and far from being aesthetically oriented. For this reason it has not been given much attention by modern Arab critics, and is often discarded as decadent. This sociopolitical trend in poetry was closely related to the fact that the post-classical age, especially under the Mamluks, was the golden age of historiography and encyclopaedic literature. It is not surprising that this period produced the "cream of thought" which is, according to the words of the 15th-century historian al-Maqrīzī, the *Muqaddima* or *Prolegomena* of Ibn Khaldūn, the most original philosophical work of the Arabs, and one of the most fascinating books of world literature. Its strength and originality lay in its focus on social history and social philosophy.

This development, however, did not free the art of poetry from the latent virus of mannerism. Word plays and intricate constructions of rhymes with interlacing and symmetrical word arrangements continued to be features of later Arabic poetry.

ORIGINALITY

The distinction drawn in Arabic literature and literary criticism between form and content has been identified by Von Grunebaum as a detriment to true poetic creativity. Medieval Arab critics concentrated their energies on formal details and virtuosity rather than on the originality of meaning.[225] He attributes this tendency to the impact of Aristotelian thought on Arabic culture; Platonic concepts, which view form and content as a unity and good and beautiful as identical, would have done more to encourage a truly creative attitude. Nicholson, however, gives a different view of this phenomenon; referring to a text of literary criticism by Thaʿālibī, he writes:

> . . . the reader will easily perceive that the chief merits of poetry were then considered to lie in elegant expression, subtle combination of words, fanciful imagery, witty conceits, and a striking use of rhetorical figures. Such indeed, are the views which prevail to this day throughout the whole Muhammadan world, and it is unreasonable to denounce them as false simply because they do not square with ours. Who shall decide when nations disagree?[226]

Von Grunebaum's opinion that Arab thinkers did not value creativity and that their interest lay mainly in formal aspects has recently been challenged by Abu-Deeb who provides many instances, particularly from the work of ʿAbd al-Qāhir al-Jurjānī, that suggest the contrary. Jurjānī's great innovation was to formulate the inseparability of meaning, imagery, and the syntactic structure as components of poetry. He viewed imagery as a form of thought integrally related to linguistic structure, and he equated the structure of the image with the essence of the meaning. He expected the intelligent poet (as opposed to the incompetent poet) to be capable of reasoning and imaginative thinking.[227]

Basically, however, in accordance with Ashʿarism—which conceives the world as finite, created by God out of nothing, to which nothing can be added—the poet's role was not to create, but to elaborate. As Heinrichs writes, invention was basically discovery.[228] Originality implied not the unlimited freedom of invention, but rather the skill to find variations on and reinterpretations of a traditional theme. The poet was expected to work within the framework of the literary tradition that goes back to pre-Islamic times.[229] De Bruyne writes of medieval European thought that ideas were measured not by the originality of their goals, but rather by their transmission of ancient established common sense.[230]

If restrictions were set on conceptual creativity, fantasy was free to achieve the highest effects in wording. Arabic classical literature, basically hostile to fictive and fantastic narration, made great use of fantastic hyperbolic descriptions. The fantastic was confined to the methods of expression which ultimately had to be based on reality.[231] From the Arabic aesthetic viewpoint, the creativity and esprit of the artist is manifest in his skill in playing with variations on a familiar theme, and in toying with allusions, innuendoes, and reminiscences. The more familiar the theme, the more interesting and difficult the artistic interpretation and variation will be. The Arab hearer or reader of a poem waits to see how the poet will treat the familiar theme, like the spectator at an opera whose expectations are focused not on the subject, but on the style of the performance. Because they are so full of allusions, many poems can be fully grasped only by an audience steeped in the Arab poetic heritage. "Intertextuality" or literary allusions and reinterpretation of familiar motifs contribute to the artistic effect.[232] As Bencheikh puts it, "The poem is the place of re-encounter between the artist and the audience."[233] There was, in a sense, also a continuous dialogue and discourse with the masters of the past, whose tradition was thus kept alive.

ʿAbd al-Qāhir al-Jurjānī stressed the importance of originality, referring to the intelligent artist (*ṣanīʿ*) as the *imām* of his craft, whose inventions and innovations (*al-bidaʿ allatī yakhtariʿuhā*) are acknowledged as superior. The art (*ṣanʿa*) he creates, with the support of divine power, is imitated by his successors and he is acknowledged as the source.[234]

The significance of originality is documented in frequent literary references to uniqueness, innovation, and first occurrences. There is also a literary genre dealing with innovations in various fields such as fashion, lifestyle, and warfare, documenting the names of persons who introduced new ideas or styles.

Ibdāʿ is a term referring to creation in the divine sense; *badīʿ* (its adjectival noun when used in the active sense meaning creator) is an attribute of God. In the classic Abbasid age, however, still under the impact of Muʿtazilism, when the idea of human creativity was not yet rejected, the term *ibdāʿ* was also used to refer to the creativity of a poet or artist. In their musical and poetic symposiums the Abbasid caliphs often used this term to praise their artists. In orthodox theology the term *bidʿa* (innovation) refers to ideas or practices that are not documented at the time of the Prophet and are thus equivalent to wrongdoings. However, the term *badīʿ* was also applied to refer to a modernistic style of literary artifices created in the 9th century and used for centuries thereafter. In the post-classical period the *ʿilm al-badīʿ* (science of *badīʿ*) was a branch of rhetoric created by al-Sakkākī (d. 1229) that deals with stylistic embellishments.[235] According to Sakkākī's theory, rhetoric consists of concept, presentation, and stylistic embellishment.

Plagiarism was severely condemned. The negative association of plagiarism is demonstrated by its Arabic name *sariqa*, which refers to the capital crime of theft, for which Islamic law applies the penalty of cutting off a hand. There is a whole literature on plagiarism which shows that while the notion of originality existed, it was different from the modern one. Taking from tradition was not wrong, but it was wrong to copy from contemporaries without giving them credit.[236] The *Book of Songs* is full of references to controversies and anecdotes about singers, composers, and poets being offended over the circulation of their melodies and the adoption of their style without credit.

The seriousness attached to the crime of plagiarism is demonstrated in the twenty third *maqāma* of al-Ḥarīrī, which deals with a quarrel between two persons concerning the theft of a poem and the eventual interference of the ruler in this quarrel. In this episode the victim of the theft says that stealing an idea is worse than stealing silver and gold, and is equivalent to stealing the soul. He adds that a poet is more eager to defend his ideas than his daughter's virginity!

IMAGINATION

Because of Aristotle's influence, the subject of imagination and its poetic implication was of interest not only to literary critics, but to the philosophers as well. Following Aristotle's *Poetics,* the philosophers al-Rāzī, al-Farābī, and Ibn Sīnā and the critics ʿAbd al-Qāhir al-Jurjānī and Ḥāzim al-Qarṭājannī emphasized the role of imagination in the poetic creation.

According to Aristotle, it is the mimetic arts of poetry, music, and dance that display the human potential. Poetry was therefore valued over the writing of history because its significance was universal rather than tied to individual events.[237] For al-Rāzī, the speech that moves the heart with pleasure should be not straight and informative, but rather poetically playful, exciting the recipient by concealing and revealing things at the same time; poetry should have emotional power.[238] Farābī tried to combine Aristotle's thoughts on poetics and on psychology by including imagination in the poetic process.[239] The objective of poetry was to move by emotive rather than intellectual means, speaking truths to the heart through imagery.[240] To him the evocative power of poetic imagery is a form of non-literal representation which, in its own way, can be truthful.[241] The imaginative power reorganizes the perceived image in a new creative combination that is not necessarily identical with the original. Farābī, however, viewed poetry not as the agent of mere aesthetic pleasure, but as a means of improving the faculty of reason and of moderating base instincts and feelings.

Ibn Rushd looks to Aristotle for inspiration when comparing historiography with poetry. Historical narration, he concludes, may contain a great deal of invented material. By contrast, poetry expresses universal truths, which are then shaped in accordance with the systematic rules of metrics. Poetry is therefore closer to philosophy than is historical narration, but it should not try to play the role of rhetoric; it should rather imitate life with color and vividness. If the poet uses the methods of reasoning, he sins against his art.[242] This approach differs from European scholastic thought, which listed poetics among the rhetorical disciplines and, as a result, did not conceive of poetry as capable of reaching the essence of things in a way inaccessible to rational thinking.[243]

The Ikhwān al-Ṣafā speak of imagination as an intellectual power that allows one to see things that no longer exist or things that have never existed, such as a camel on top of a tree, a tree growing on the back of a camel, a bird with four legs, a winged horse, or an ass with a human face. Imagination is needed for craftsmanship, for the craftsman imagines the object before beginning to fashion it.[244] With the power of imagination human beings can wander from east to west, over land and sea, across mountains and plains, and through the firmament. They can see the beginning and the end of the world, real and unreal things.[245] The Ikhwān al-Ṣafā attributed to all skills and crafts a common basis in this imaginative power.

Ibn Sīnā recognized the need for poetic embellishment such as that produced by rhyme, but added that this alone did not suffice to produce poetry, which needs images to reach the heart and the imagination. The highest aesthetic effect is produced by the virtuosity of the artist with images or the poet with words in order to represent the world in new, unexplored ways.

> The imaginative is the speech to which the soul yields, accepting and rejecting matters without pondering, reasoning or choice. In brief, it corresponds psychologically rather than ratiocinatively.[246]

> Human beings are more amenable to imaginative representation than to conviction.

> Imaginative assent... is a compliance due to the wonder and pleasure that are caused by the utterance itself.[247]

Ibn Sīnā considered the poet's creativity to be unlimited because the means of poetic representation are neither limited nor fixed. A comparison of the beloved with the moon may not be literally accurate, but it is true insofar as it conveys an idea of beauty. The role of the poet is to reveal truth by inventing telling images; the indirect language of poetry is thus a means of expressing truth.[248] Ibn Sīnā also acknowledged that the brilliance of striking and impressive literary images was a source of pleasure.[249]

ʿAbd al-Qāhir al-Jurjānī attributed the power of poetic imagery to its ability to penetrate hidden meanings and thus reveal invisible things. Image had a power similar to magic; it can "join east with west," "show life in the lifeless," "unify the opposites," "blend life with death and water with fire," and it can "sweeten the bitter" and "beautify the ugly."[250] Veiled poetic speech invites the recipient to search for the hidden pearl; it is this quest rather than direct rational speech that stimulates pleasure.[251]

Ḥāzim al-Qarṭājannī (d. 1285) was one of the most original of the literary critics, although his influence was not far-reaching. He attributed to image the power of transcending things and manipulating their qualities by turning beautiful to ugly and vice-versa. The image is by its nature more powerful than the original, because it is based on condensation and on new associations. Poetry furthermore differs from scientific knowledge, with its complex system of theoretical thinking, in that it hits the senses directly; it is like a glass which reveals its content immediately to the eye.[252] Ḥāzim emphasized the poetic link between imagination and emotion; images produced by the poet's imagination strike and stimulate the recipient's own imagination and thus arouse emotion. He understood image in the sense of Ibn Sīnā, as the mental apprehension of the real object. This view of the image as a psychological, not merely a visual, phenomenon adds a new dimension to poetry, giving it a more autonomous function than that of faithfully reproducing in words the mere visual or descriptive content of an image. As Ibn al-Haytham had done earlier with visual perception, Ḥāzim recognized the psychological depth in poetic perception.

This discourse of the philosophers and literary critics on imagination and its creative role did not, however, imply that artists or poets were seen as the recipients of supernatural powers. They remained human beings working at the cultivation of their own talents and potential.

The Visual Arts

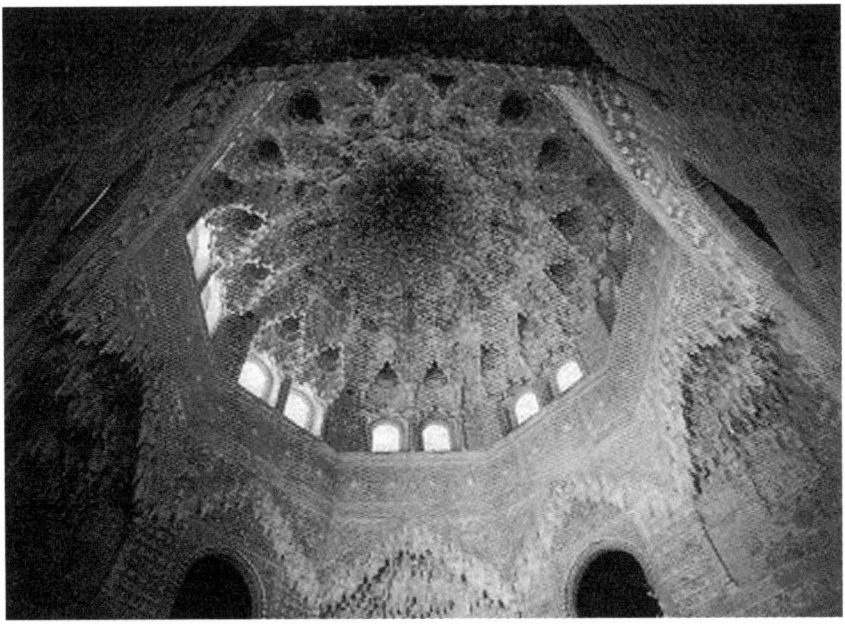

Muqarnas ceiling in the Hall of the Two Sisters in the Alhambra, 14th c.

The Status of the Arts

The principle that any art or science is based on learning and skill rather than genius and inspiration is rooted in Islamic orthodoxy and its stress on the unique and exclusive character of the Koran's revelation to the Prophet. Once Islam had denied that poets had supernatural creative faculties and thereby ended the champion role they played in pre-Islamic society, skill and practice necessarily became the major sources of excellence, not only in poetry but in other disciplines as well. The philosophers agreed with the theologians on this point, rejecting the Neoplatonic principle that views the artist as the recipient of a vision, or metaphysical idea. Ibn Rushd, citing Aristotle, described art as nothing more than the material form of an object produced in the artist's mind.[253]

For Ibn Sīnā it is the human fantasy alone that selects and composes images of objects never seen, without the intermediary of demonic or supernatural agents.[254] In his theories of perception, mental powers are categorized in a sequence of intellectual levels beginning with the simplest, apprehension through the senses, and culminating in the most complex, conceptual thinking. Sensory perception occurs through the abstraction of forms by means of an image (*ṣūra*) in the brain. This is followed by a perceptual analysis of the significance of the image, which is accomplished through the inner power of the brain. The information thus received acquires significance after it has gone through a process of selection, comparison, and association with other experiences collected in the memory. Complex and abstract ideas are produced by association and generalization of images collected in the memory and representing empirical data. The human soul can by itself attain the first degrees of perception related to sensation, imagination, and judgment, i.e., the faculties used in mundane human activities. Whereas intellectual perfection is a matter of personal endeavor,[255] the highest degrees of abstraction or conceptualization can be reached only with the help of the active intellect, which is a separate intelligence, a kind of intermediary, between the human and the divine.

For Ibn Sīnā, as for Farābī, the highest stage of human reason, or creative thinking, is that which leads, with the assistance of the active intellect, to the faculty of prophecy. Farābī thought of imagination as a form of creative thinking in which prophecy is also rooted. The source of this power, however, originates in the soul, which earns the support of the active intellect only after having achieved the full apprehension of the intelligible world.[256] After having attained this high degree of lucidity through the laborious cultivation of its intellectual faculties, the soul is able to receive the enlightenment that allows it to apprehend intuitively.[257] The prophets, by rising above and detaching themselves from the level of worldly concerns, attain this extraordinary form of cognition. All other creative activities remain rooted in the worldly sphere. In Farābī's ideal city, poets, writers, and intellectuals occupy only an intermediate position below the philosopher-prophet and above the masses.

Philosophy and sufism, likewise, associated superior intuitive intelligence only with prophecy and sainthood, that is, exclusively with religion. Poets or artists could lay no claim to it. This view is consistent with the orthodox rationalistic interpretation of the poet's and any other artist's role. It diverges from Neoplatonism, which attributes to the artist a divinatory or revelatory function. In the Neoplatonic doctrine of emanation, divine light connects the celestial and the earthly realms, bestowing form and beauty on all things; the artist's role is to reveal the relationship between visible and invisible beauty, and artistic creation is thus part of the divine creation.

According to Ghazālī, supernatural powers are involved only in religious revelation. He mentioned revelation and inspiration as a source of spiritual knowledge, revelation (*waḥiyy*) being a prerogative of prophets and inspiration (*ilhām*) of mystics. Mystics, by freeing themselves from the bondage of the flesh, are able to receive the divine gift of supernatural power. *Waḥiyy* is a higher form of inspiration, distinct from the profane scholarly knowledge acquired through study. Although Ghazālī does not say it explicitly, the arts belong to the latter. Poets' or artists' work is not a form of revelation, but a manifestation of their skill and knowledge. The case of the Koranic revelation is very different and it is unique. As the highest form of literary expression, the Koran was revealed to the illiterate Prophet in his function as messenger of God through a vision, without any personal contribution on his part.

The "demythologising" of the poet in Islam was paralleled by similar rationalistic approaches to other disciplines. Architecture was not idealized as a superior creative art as it was by Plato and Aristotle.[258] One of the arguments used against figural representation was that the artist should not imitate God's work, because playing the role of creator would be blasphemy.[259]

In Ghazālī's conception, the work of art reflected the greatness of the artist in the same way that the beauty of the universe reflected that of the Creator. Although he draws a parallel between the two forms of creation, Ghazālī does not attribute a divine source to artistic production. God gave human beings the means to adorn themselves—to produce objects for aesthetic purposes—and they need God's help in all their endeavors, but man-made beauty is a mundane matter not associated with a divine source. God speaks to humanity directly through the Koran and indirectly through the mediation of the prophets. He does not specifically address the artist or craftsman. Despite his allegiance to Ashʿarī principles, Ghazālī, following Ibn Sīnā and anticipating St. Thomas Aquinas, separates human work from divine creation, thus giving it an autonomous character. God's power over all things does not imbue the artist's work with divine qualities.

Ibn Khaldūn lived and worked at a time when historiography was a major form of cultural expression. His own philosophy of history and social evolution was concerned with the phenomenon of civilization and its decline. He was interested in epistemology and concrete reality; he rejected metaphysical and speculative philosophy. His sober and down-to-earth mind is representative of Arabic culture of the post-classical age, which ultimately refuted speculative as well as esoteric thinking. His view that the arts cannot flourish outside prosperous urban and cultural environments leaves no room for sacral or metaphysical associations with the arts. For Ibn Khaldūn, humankind is born ignorant, and knowledge is the basis of all sciences. Sciences and crafts are the product of reasoning, which distinguishes people from animals. Physical as well as intellectual and imaginative activities are rooted in the material world, that is, in the brain, and can, therefore, be perfected. Knowledge needs continuity and accumulation to progress; otherwise it wanes, leading to the decline of the arts and sciences. In order to be effective, science has to be rooted in a long tradition. "The move from energy to action does not occur at once, in particular as far the arts and crafts are concerned; it therefore needs time." Once it is perfected and refined, knowledge will in turn stimulate and improve the intelligence.[260]

In Ibn Khaldūn's view, knowledge derives from perceptions of the brain and the body; we gain practical experience with the aid of our senses. Knowledge that is based on experience is sounder than knowledge based on mere information. All sciences and crafts have to be learned through experience, whether they are theoretically or practically oriented, for experience educates and enlightens. Writing and arithmetic (*kitāba, ḥisāb*) are among the most didactic crafts.[261] God has made the human being His representative on earth because only humans, among all creatures, have minds capable of systematic empirical as well as theoretical thinking. Ibn Khaldūn thus makes clear that intelligence itself is not a matter of pure nature; rather it is a skill that can be improved and perfected by education and training. The city dweller is superior to the bedouin, not because their nature is different, but because an urban upbringing endows one with higher qualifications.

Ibn Khaldūn comments on the philosophical theory of perception, which he as an orthodox Muslim rejects. Imagination is part of the brain's activity and operates with images perceived by the senses, processing them and storing them in memory or displaying them in dreams. It is the material mind that creates the symbols we see in our dreams, such as an enemy symbolized by the sea, evil by a snake, a woman by a vessel. Ibn Khaldūn agrees that human perception consists of a corporeal and a spiritual level, but both are centered in the human brain, which is physical, not metaphysical. The spiritual experience of the sufi is equally rooted in the activities of the brain, including memory and imagination.[262] When it comes to the conflict between religion and philosophy, however, he rejects the philosophers' approach, which excludes revelation; that view blurs the lines between the material and the immaterial, disregarding the magnitude of the universe and excluding the divine power. He agrees with Ghazālī that rational thinking can sharpen the mind, but cannot bring the supreme happiness promised by religion.

Human beings acquire knowledge through a process of experience and learning; they are not born with it. The brain is the center that processes and integrates sensory perceptions. Perception is not a product of direct contact with the objects, but an outcome of the integrating process of the brain.[263] Thought is contingent upon the material functions of the brain.

Knowledge was highly valued not only for its moral and religious function, but also for the pleasure it conveys, which could even have a physical dimension comparable to that of erotic pleasure.[264] This hedonist approach can also be perceived in Ghazālī's words when he writes that the soul, which seeks truth, finds delight in learning even trifling subjects, such as playing chess. The higher the subject matter of the knowledge obtained, however, the greater the delight. Knowledge leads to worldly happiness as well as to spiritual exaltation and ultimately to God.

Abū Ḥayyān al-Tawḥīdī qualifies knowledge as useful because of the information it provides to ease the problems of life and enlighten the mind. It is also a source of satisfaction and entertainment that can be pursued for its own pleasure.[265] Abū Ḥayyān, who was a litterateur and compiler of philosophical statements rather than a systematic philosopher, presents contradictory notions of *ṣināʿa* (science, technique, or art) collected from various sources. On one occasion, he writes that *ṣināʿa* is human and derives from nature, which itself derives from God; it is therefore subordinate to nature and cannot be compared to the divine creation. By *ṣināʿa* Abū Ḥayyān meant activity in any field with any purpose based on mental power and requiring reflection.[266] Elsewhere, however, Abū Ḥayyān presents the idea that nature needs *ṣināʿa* to complement and perfect itself. *Sīnāʿa* derives from the intellect and the soul, and imposes itself upon nature, which is therefore subordinate to the soul. Nature loves the soul, submitting to it and abiding by its action. It needs *ṣināʿa* for its fulfillment and perfection. *Sīnāʿa*, in turn, needs nature to interact with, so that both may become complete. Using the resources of the mind and artistic excellence, the musician decks the material supplied by nature in elegant attire that makes it attractive.[267] This notion derives from Aristotle who said that matter yearns for the form to reach its perfection just as the female longs for the male.[268]

Although the Islamic arts are largely autonomous and should not be viewed as dependent on other theoretical disciplines, we should not overlook the many statements concerning poetic delectability that also deal with general aesthetic criteria and include comparisons with aspects of the visual arts. Paradoxically, of the rare literary comments to be found on visual arts, a number are on painting and sculpture, although these arts are not at the core of the Arab artistic tradition, while architecture, which was so central, is not even mentioned as an art or a science. Nor do the Arab authors elaborate on other arts and crafts so integral to their society, such as pottery or metalwork. Various texts praise the illusory or *trompe-l'oeil* effects that painting or sculpture can produce.[269] Whenever Arab historians describe pre-Islamic or non-Islamic sculpture and painting, such as gifts sent by foreign monarchs, they grow enthusiastic and excited about the illusionist character of these objects. The Ikhwān al-Ṣafā make an interesting observation on the art of painting that reveals non-Islamic ideas. They relate how an artist made a gorgeous painting with magnificent colors, which everyone admired until another artist came along with a piece of charcoal and painted a black man so vividly that he seemed to be pointing his finger at the spectators. Immediately the spectators shifted attention to the second artist's work, abandoning the colorful painting in favor of the sober but more vivid and expressive one.[270]

The comparisons between poetry and painting made by Arabic philosophers and literary critics, notwithstanding the predominantly aniconic character of their own artistic tradition, can be explained by the Greek influence. Farābī wrote:

> Now we may say that there is a certain relationship between the practitioners of this art [poetry] and painters; one might almost say that the materials of their crafts differ, but their forms, their activities, their intentions are the same, or at least that they are similar. The art of poetry operates with words, the art of painting with colours, and therein they differ; but in practice both produce likenesses, and both aim at impressing men's imaginations and senses with imitations.[271]

Similarly, ʿAbd al-Qāhir al-Jurjānī:

> Careful craftsmanship and skilful artistic creation in the images [of poetry] which charm and appeal to the hearers, and in the imaginative analogies and conceits which excite the patrons, have an effect on the soul similar to the effect of beholding images composed by skilful artists in drawing, painting, carving and sculpture. Just as the latter arouse admiration and delight, and impart to the soul when it encounters them visually a fresh

experience unknown to it before, and imbue it with a kind of magic whose value and significance none can deny or ignore (and you no doubt know what the case is with idols, and the state of mind of their worshippers who glorify them and are totally charmed by them), so it is with poetry in respect to the images which it creates, the invention which it formulates, and the ideas which it instills into the soul . . .[272]

The Arabs inherited the classification of sciences from the Greeks and adapted it to their own culture by including religious sciences, history, and practical mathematics. Some lists, such as those of the Ikhwān al-Ṣafā and al-ʿĀmirī, include manual crafts (*ḥiraf*) as well.[273] Whereas the Greek classification reflects aristocratic thinking that acknowledges only mental activities and disregards manual work, the Arabs included in their repertoire of sciences a number of practical disciplines, such as pharmacology, which they added to medicine; almanacs, which they added to geography; and the arithmetic of inheritance, tax calculation, commercial transactions, and various other bureaucratic crafts, which they added to Greek arithmetic. The Islamization of the Greek sciences in Arabic culture elevated the practical disciplines to a higher status.[274] Arithmetic was highly valued; all authors emphasize its pedagogic significance and its usefulness in all aspects of human activities, though architecture, in the sense of creative design, is not included among them. Rebstock remarks that it is rarely mentioned in mathematical literature and then only vaguely and merely as an aspect of applied geometry. Texts dealing with the mensuration (*misāḥa*) of dome and *muqarnas* surfaces and the calculation of architectural volumes were supposed to serve cost calculations for administrative purposes rather than for design, or perhaps were merely a mental exercise.[275]

Arabic thought did not follow the classic distinction between liberal and mechanical arts as higher and lower crafts, although a clear distinction was made between theory and practice within the same discipline. In biographical literature, for example, it was always noted in a physician's qualifications whether he was a better practitioner or scholar. The same discrimination was made in the field of music. Although the Arabs did not believe in principle that manual labor was inferior, the *Arabian Nights* usually depict the artisan as wretchedly poor, unlike the merchant.

Farābī, particularly, emphasized the practical aspects of knowledge in all disciplines, from philosophy to music. He wrote:

> The end of the theoretical is truth and knowledge simply. The end of the practical is choosing one thing and avoiding another. Human beings do not attain the end of the practical part through their own insights, but through knowledge of it that precedes or is simultaneous with action. On the other hand, when a person attains knowledge of it without acting, then that knowledge is in vain.[276]

He distinguished between experimental knowledge that arises from the practice of an art and knowledge reached through mere learning and reasoning. Some arts are essentially theoretical, others more practical, which in modern terminology would be expressed as the difference between science and technology. Information based on the practical crafts is not uniform or predictable, as it derives from random individual cases.[277]

In Arabic literary sources the term *ṣanaʿa* (to make, to produce) and *ṣināʿa* (craft, science, art) are used for all sciences, arts, and crafts, whether practical or theoretical, religious or profane. They are applied to the poet, the historian, the musician, the physician, the theologian, the calligrapher, the peasant. Rhetoric is as much a *ṣināʿa* or craft as jewelry-making or goldsmithing. All equally require learning and practice, intelligence and skill in mastering the tools. All those involved in a *ṣināʿa* have to polish and sort out their material to produce the required effect. Even human character has to be educated and perfected.[278]

According to the Ikhwān al-Ṣafā, to practice an art with perfection is an act of allegiance and devotion to God, for there is a *ḥadīth* that says that God loves the skillful craftsman (*inna 'llāha yuḥibbu 'l-ṣāniʿ al-ḥādhiq*), because He Himself is the wise and perfect artisan. To practice an art with excellence brings man closer to God, for He is the perfect maker and He loves the excellent craftsman.[279] Perhaps under the impact of Stoic thought, which distinguishes between necessary crafts and crafts for pleasure,[280] the Ikhwān al-Ṣafā categorized the arts and crafts according to their usefulness and necessity, a principle that was adopted centuries later by Ibn Khaldūn. Husbandry, building, tailoring, and waste disposal belong to the essential and useful crafts. Crafts that deal with beauty and ornamentation, such as silk, perfume, or jewelry-making, are luxurious. Some rely for their importance on valuable material; others consist essentially of skill.[281]

Ibn Khaldūn describes husbandry using the same term (*ṣināʿa*) that he uses for music. For him the bookbinder is as important as the author because both are equally necessary for the production and propagation of literature. He draws a distinction between the basic crafts that are vital for securing food and lodging and the more sophisticated and luxurious ones. Elegance, refinement and ornament are manifestations of affluence and products of urban civilization. Music, book-making, rope-dancing, architectural decoration, and other decorative crafts belong to such forms of refinement.[282] Ibn Khaldūn also distinguishes between simple knowledge or information and complex knowledge or science. In urban or civilized societies any science (*ʿilm*) is a craft or profession (*ṣināʿa*), with its own rules and systems that have to be studied. In simple bedouin societies *ʿilm* (which in this context includes religion) is merely orally communicated information. Scientific learning or study differs from simple knowledge.[283]

Not all skills and techniques had corresponding sciences or theoretical bases, as medicine, music, and calligraphy did. Architecture and the decorative arts had none and in the theoretical sciences the lines between disciplines were flexible. In the practical professions, however, the division of labor was pronounced.[284] Like their Greek counterparts, Arabic philosophers or religious scholars worked in various disciplines simultaneously, combining theology with medicine and astronomy, but a dyer would dye only in blue, not in red. With the exception of calligraphy, no written rules exist for any of the visual arts that would bestow on them the status of a discipline. Unlike poetry, which was controlled by a very articulate literary criticism, and unlike music, which had its own forum, there was no such thing as criticism of the visual arts.

Although Arabic theorists put theory on an equal footing with practice, a difference in status was drawn between the arts that were based on theoretical disciplines and those that were practical. Owing to the segregation between the craftsman and the scholar, the arts that were only practical were ignored in the historical literature. Although poets and literary critics were fond of referring to the jeweler's art as the model for the poet, no jewelers are documented in historical or biographical sources. There are occasional references to calligraphers or illuminators, but they are rather accidental and do not always correspond to the artistic importance of the persons mentioned. Many artists whose influence was significant were not even recorded.

In some texts the higher pursuit of knowledge was opposed to the lower pursuit of action. The reality of economics, which dictates its own rules, was demonstrated by Bīrūnī, who referred to "the difference between knowledge and practical work" in rock carving. He pointed out that the artist whose function was to select the rock crystals and to design their carving pattern earned a much higher salary than the craftsman who did the actual carving.[285] Rāghib al-Iṣfahānī (12th century) esteemed activities based on the intellect higher than those based on the senses, because of the intellect's superiority.[286]

Whereas in poetry and music the authorship of a work, even the composition of an individual variation, was recorded, and artistic property defended against attempts at plagiarism, the craftsman had no such recognition. Although Arabic historians were eager to record the first occurrences of something in many aspects of life and culture, artisanal and architectural innovation were not thus noted. The visual arts were seen rather as collective achievements, as they were in many other pre-modern cultures.

Manual work was not despised, however, and some intellectuals or religious scholars even practiced crafts, albeit as a second choice. They are recorded in biographical literature as scholars who mastered a craft, rather than as craftsmen with an academic education. Without their scholarly qualifications, they would not have been mentioned. One of the Mamluk sultans, al-Ṣāliḥ Ṣalāḥ al-Dīn (1351–54) of the Qalāwūn dynasty, used to take private lessons in the art of silk-making and other crafts. The first caliphs and companions of the Prophet were associated with crafts, the caliphs Abū Bakr and ʿUthmān Ibn ʿAffān had been weavers; ʿAmr Ibn al-ʿĀṣ, the conqueror of Egypt, was a butcher; Saʿd Ibn Waqqās, who conquered Iran and Central Asia, was an arrow-maker. The guilds in the late medieval period chose for their patrons Muslim saints who had also been craftsmen.

Geographers and urban historians measured the glory of cities partly in terms of the crafts they produced. It is difficult, however, to estimate exactly how highly valued the craftsman involved in artistic work may have been. Although the scarcity of information in this regard is suggestive, the occasional presence of craftsmen's signatures on art objects shows that artists did take pride in their work. There were, of course, individual cases of art patronage which brought forth exceptional achievements, as the case of the Fatimid vizier al-Yāzūrī who organized a contest between two painters, an Egyptian and an Iraqi, to depict female dancers on murals using *trompe-l'oeil* effects.[287] The artists and the craftsmen, like the poets of the classical period, were generously rewarded by the rulers with money and robes of honor. The Mamluk architect and master-mason Aḥmad al-Ṭūlūnī, for example, began his career in the building trades as head of the stonecutters and masons, probably also as a contractor, and managed to become an amir, in spite of his non-Mamluk origin. Eventually Sultan Barqūq twice married into al-Ṭūlūnī's family. His descendents continued to control the building craft for decades.[288]

An Egyptian tale in the *Arabian Nights*, the tale of Qamar al-Zamān, includes a short but revealing illustration of the meaning of a work of art. A jeweler was commissioned to produce an outstanding piece of jewelry; when he began work on it he left his shop and went home to work for two reasons: first, he did not want to be seen by his apprentices, so they could not copy his work; second, he wanted to have his beloved wife near him while he worked, for her appearance inspired him to create jewelry worthy of kings.[289] This episode illustrates two aspects of an artist's work: the subjective emotional part that responds to stimulation and inspiration, and the physical part that requires skill and can be imitated by any sufficiently trained person.

Ibn al-Razzāz al-Jazarī, the author of a famous illustrated book on mechanical devices, was a maker of automata before writing his book in the first decade of the 13th century.[290] His patron, the Urtukid sultan of Diyārbakr Maḥmūd Qarā Arslān, assigned him the task of writing down all he knew about making mechanical devices so that his achievements could be saved for posterity. The fear that his knowledge might be lost shows that the practitioners' procedures and techniques were usually not written down, but rather transmitted through apprenticeship. In the case of a sophisticated and precarious craft such as that of automata-making, royal patronage was essential for the realization of a book on the subject. Jazarī's name has been recorded by posterity because of the book's illustrations, which became famous and were repeatedly copied. Little is known about the fate of the automata themselves. Jazarī's book, written in the first person, describes his research and practical work step by step, referring to the difficulties that confronted him and boasting of the originality of his work and its success, though not neglecting to give credit to his sources and predecessors. His descriptions of the automata are extremely detailed. "Any scientific knowledge that is not verified by practice," he wrote, "remains uncertain, [somewhere] between right and wrong."[291]

Jazarī is also the author of a rare craftsman's document which describes systematically and in detail the production of a bronze door for a royal palace. His tasks included both the casting of the metal and the decoration of the door surface with geometrical stars. Jazarī praises his door as a valuable object of unparalleled beauty, a *durra yatīma* (unique pearl). As in his automata book, he speaks as a learned craftsman rather than as what we would call today an artist; his interest lies in technique rather than in the design or aesthetic effect.

The philosophers and literary critics who associated poetry with imagination and compared it with painting did not mention the builder or the decorator in this context. Nor were potters and metalworkers ever mentioned in literary sources, in spite of their significant contribution to Islamic art. The monuments of past cultures were viewed as the achievements of societies led by powerful rulers; they either expressed the monarchs' search for immortality or documented cultural grandeur, but they were not interpreted as works of art in the sense of an idea generated in an individual's mind.

Some modern historians try to link Islamic art to theological or sufi doctrines, although there is not any literary evidence to justify this link. On the contrary, everything seems to indicate that the ulema did not involve themselves in reflection on the visual arts or in discourse with craftsmen. Unlike European medieval art, which can be described as religious art, the impact of religious thought on Islamic art is unclear. The scarcity of figural motifs can be explained by religious doctrines, but a direct influence of Muslim thought on the arabesque and the geometrical star cannot be determined. It remains a matter of speculation and leaves modern historians with conflicting interpretations. This does not, however, preclude that there are always links, however indirect, among the various cultural manifestations of a society.

Light, which occupies a more prominent place than any other theme in the Koran as well as in philosophy, is used symbolically; but no aesthetic statements or ideas can be found in Arab thought comparable to those expressed by Abbot Suger linking light with the arts in connection with the Gothic cathedral. This is all the more astonishing when we consider how inventively and imaginatively Islamic artists produced effects with light in architecture and art objects, inventing devices such as *muqarnas* vaults, pierced screens, window grills, and magnificent lamps of enameled glass or filigreed metal. Gothic art has been connected to Neoplatonic thought and to the medieval metaphysics of light; although Neoplatonic theories of light were of equally great significance in sufi thought, their impact on the arts cannot be assessed. The golden age for the sufis in Egypt and Syria was under Mamluk rule, the period when religious authorities made the most explicit and rigorous statements against figural representations, which is probably what led to their disappearance from the Mamluk decorative arts in favor of epigraphy.[292] Elsewhere in the Muslim world, the ascendance of sufism coincided with an increasing taste for painting, which led some modern historians to see a connection. Although Mamluk sultans and Mamluk religious life were strongly under the influence of sufism, the nature of Mamluk visual arts shows nothing that can be interpreted as sufi influence. Artistic evolution followed its own line, independent of religious trends. Unlike in literature, in the visual arts Shīʿa, Sunni, or Muʿtazilit movements play no part in the formation of artistic styles. The artistic evolution in Egypt from the Sunni Tulunid rulers to the Shīʿa Fatimids and back to the Sunni Ayyubids reveals no sign of religious rupture. Similarly in Iran, the art of the Shīʿa Ṣafāvids follows that of their Sunni Timurid predecessors with no apparent stylistic break. In Islamic art, there is no phenomenon comparable to the association of Baroque architecture with Catholicism in Europe. The lack of such connections confirms the profane character of the arts and the indifference of the religious establishment toward them.

A rationalistic approach tries to make a connection between the importance of mathematics among the medieval Muslim sciences and the role of geometry in artistic design. Mathematics was acknowledged and celebrated both as a theoretical and as a practical discipline; it was even dealt with in a literary genre concerned with rarities and puzzles. Although Arabic culture gave an important place to mathematics and although geometry characterized the decorative arts, Arabic literature does not discuss the visual or aesthetic aspects of geometry. In all classifications of the sciences, geometry is described as a basic tool for a number of crafts including mensuration and building, with no reference to its artistic aspect or its application as decoration or surface treatment.[293]

In treating geometry as the basis for all disciplines, the Ikhwān al-Ṣafā were considering not its artistic application but its intellectual value. Ibn Khaldūn likewise wrote that geometry purifies the mind because it is based on clear rules that cannot fail. He praises arithmetic for its enlightening effect on the mind. It is essential to commercial transactions and calculations of inheritance and is therefore, according to the Prophet in several *ḥadīth*s, a most important discipline. Mathematics is useful for engineering, carpentry, mechanics, land surveys, and optics. He mentions building and decoration in a different context without even associating it with mathematics. There he deals with the building trade as a form of urban refinement and civilization. Ibn Khaldūn uses purely functional terms to describe this craft and the various techniques it involves. The builder should know about *handasa* (meaning here engineering) to be able to erect straight walls and aqueducts and to transfer heavy stone blocks. Building is attributed to masons and decorators. The great monuments of ancient cultures were the work of several generations. He writes in greater detail about the carpenter's work, which needs practice, adding that Euclid and Pliny had been carpenters, and Noah is the patron of this craft.[294] Abū Ḥayyān al-Tawḥīdī describes geometry as a rational science dealing with lengths, surfaces, volumes, and angles.[295] Ibn ʿArabī, with all his esoteric mysticism, refers to geometry as a discipline useful for mensuration.[296] None of these intellectuals mentions geometrical design in this context or makes any reference to the visual or artistic aspect of geometry, and no one refers to the *muqarnas* as a geometrical phenomenon or even uses this term. These writers agree with the mathematicians who, even in their manuals on applied geometry, spoke neither of architecture in terms of creative design nor of geometry in terms of aesthetic devices.

The characteristics of Arab art, mainly in ornament and surface treatment, have not been recognized or articulated in the Arabic written sources as specifically Islamic. Neither in documents nor in narrative sources can we expect to find a definition of what we know as Islamic design with its characteristic geometrical character. If some authors have described with fascination realistic paintings or sculptures from past or foreign cultures, when it comes to Islamic art, with its predilection for abstraction, they have nothing to say. Their words are vague, dealing with color, precious materials, and aesthetic effect rather than with substance. It is significant in this regard that the Arabic term used for the geometrical star design, *ḍarb khayṭ*, does not derive from mathematical literature, but comes rather from craftsmen's jargon; it means something like "thread stroke" and clearly refers to the technique of drawing the pattern. Ibn Khaldūn and Jazarī utilize this word, also used in *waqf* documents, which could not have been coined in scholarly circles, but only by craftsmen. No Arabic words expresses what is now called the arabesque; it is mentioned neither in medieval literature nor in documents. The word *muqarnas* is also not found in any classical Arabic dictionary and must also derive from craftsmen's jargon.

References to artistic works by historians are mostly subjective, demonstrating that they were entirely unaware of any theory for building or even for ornament. Those who recorded the building activities of the rulers did not discuss what a mosque should look like, nor did they associate the form of a mosque with any symbolism.

Maqrīzī, the major historian of Cairo and its monuments, conveys the aesthetic experience rather than the image of the object when describing its buildings. Of the citadel of Rawḍa he writes, "its opulent decoration is amazing, the beauty of the ceiling decoration and the unparalleled marbles are dazzling."[297] About the Ṭaybarsiyya college he writes: "most original, best shape, most pleasant presentation due to the perfection of the work and the quality of craftsmanship." The portal of al-Nāṣir's *madrasa* is "the most astounding work made by man's hand."[298] Sometimes he notices a technical tour-de-force, as the *muqarnas* in a palace made of one piece, or the prayer hall in Sultan Ḥasan's mosque that boasts the largest vault in the world.[299] He never refers to geometry, arabesque, or even calligraphy.

This absence of abstract definition for Islamic design illustrates the gap between the intellectual and the practical domains. The craftsmen who drew the geometric star had no aesthetic theories; the historian was not informed about the craftsmen's techniques. Even an author like Jazarī, who was familiar with Greek mathematics and therefore not a simple craftsman, attributes no higher meaning to the geometrical design of his door. It is one of the techniques he has mastered, no different from others, such as the casting of the bronze.

A text attributed to the philosopher and physician al-Rāzī that refers to the significance of mural paintings in public baths is often cited in discussions of figural motifs in Islamic culture. Al-Rāzī observed that the painted scenes had tonic powers, but probably the craftsmen who painted them were themselves unaware that the ancient sages had selected their themes according to certain criteria, with specific associations serving specific purposes.[300] This observation shows that the artist was not expected to be intellectually trained, and that the philosopher or intellectual knew more about the artistic work than did the artist himself.

In Mamluk Cairo the designers (*rassāmīn)* who drew the patterns for embroidery and brocades were established in a market named to them and located in the city's commercial center.[301] Most likely the work of these designers was not confined to textile patterns, but must have served other techniques as well, since textile patterns are also found in other crafts. Unlike the calligraphers who must have worked in the chancery or in an academic institution, the artists and craftsmen belonged in the marketplace, even when their main customer was the court.

That treatises on applied geometry and mechanics existed does not mean that they were utilized by the builders. Almanac literature was not used by farmers, but was aimed at a scholarly audience;[302] al-Kindī's and Farābī's books on music were not written for musicians, but mainly for scholars. Authors such as Ibn al-Haytham and Buzjānī, who dealt with building as a form of applied geometry and wrote treatises in this subject, were not themselves practitioners of the building crafts, and we do not know yet of any Muslim builder who wrote treatises based on his own experience. These studies, like other products of the classical Abbasid age such as mathematical games and the Banū Mūsā's book on mechanical devices, were of academic interest. They reflect the universal curiosity of this period, which extended to the vernacular and even the vulgar. Books on building technology are sometimes mentioned in the biographies of late Mamluk scholars, together with Euclid's geometry or Galen's medicine, among the literature that any erudite scholar was familiar with. Arabic biographical dictionaries tell a great deal about scholars who read books and acquired their *ijāza* (a certificate allowing the student to teach a particular work) without utilizing this knowledge in practice. The medical scholar and the professional physician in the post-classical Arab world went their separate ways;[303] building and architecture were similarly divided. The recognition of the value of practice does not imply that the relationship between theory and practice was necessarily always intimate; it could be indirect.[304]

The application of geometry in craftsmanship was an outgrowth of a culture that valued the mathematical sciences and, most of all, made them available to a large group. The inclination to mathematical and exact sciences alone does not explain the essence of Islamic design. Greek culture developed these sciences and yet Greek art took a very different direction. Medieval Europe was also fascinated by geometry and the symbolism of numbers, as is manifest in Gothic art, as the Renaissance considered mathematics to be the basic for all forms of art.

About the Gothic period, Le Goff writes that architects were perhaps the only technicians who enjoyed high recognition and prestige. The art of architecture became a science and architects acquired an academic aura; like scholars, they were allowed to use title "master." In France, learned architects elevated themselves above the level of the architect-craftsman, whereas in Italy the situation was different; they remained building practitioners.[305] It is possible that this was also the case in the post-classical Muslim world. The architect who designed the Taj Mahal may have been a mathematician, but the notion of a scientist-architect does not exist in the Arabic-speaking world. The design of Mamluk mosques in Cairo or Merinid *madrasa*s in Fez lacked the aura of scientific achievement. The persons involved in the building crafts carried the title *muʿallim*, which was applied only to a practitioner and would not have been used for a scholar.[306]

The Significance of Artistic Beauty

God created the world and ornamented *(zayyana)* it. He created the universe with the potential, and man with the ability, to produce devices of embellishment. The word *zīna* means ornament as well as beauty, including moral beauty. In Arabic aesthetic perception, beauty is not purely functional and plain, but rather crafted, elaborate, and ornate. Not the material alone in its simplicity, but the work added to it qualifies anything as beautiful. Accordingly, elegance and refinement are attributes of artistic beauty.

Undecorated objects are rare in Islamic art; even cheap objects bear some kind of ornament, as Ettinghausen noted.[307] In the *Encyclopaedia of Islam*, Islamic art is defined as an "art of decorators and ornamenters,"[308] which is certainly too narrow a definition to withstand scholarly scrutiny, but it does convey the effect Islamic art has on Westerners. Western philosophers understood ornament as a means of enhancement through the addition of unessential details: "It is always applied to a pre-existing structure and never exists on its own."[309] In Arabic culture, ornament is an essential attribute of beauty. Abū 'l-ʿAlā' al-Maʿarrī, moaning Aleppo's loss in the death of a great intellectual, said that the city was now without "anklet or bracelet," meaning without culture.[310] For something to be without ornament was equivalent to its being barren or desolate. The Arabic word *zayyana* means both to embellish and to produce a beautiful thing, as God embellished the heavens with stars.

Ornament was considered a component of music. In his *Great Book of Music* al-Farābī emphasized the aesthetic function of musical ornament as adding brilliance, elegance, grandeur, and opulence. The distinction he makes between basic and ornamental notes is interesting because it describes ornament as an essential constituent without which the object is not complete:

> Every melody consists of two types of notes. The first type is equivalent to the warp and woof in a cloth, or mud bricks and wood in buildings. The

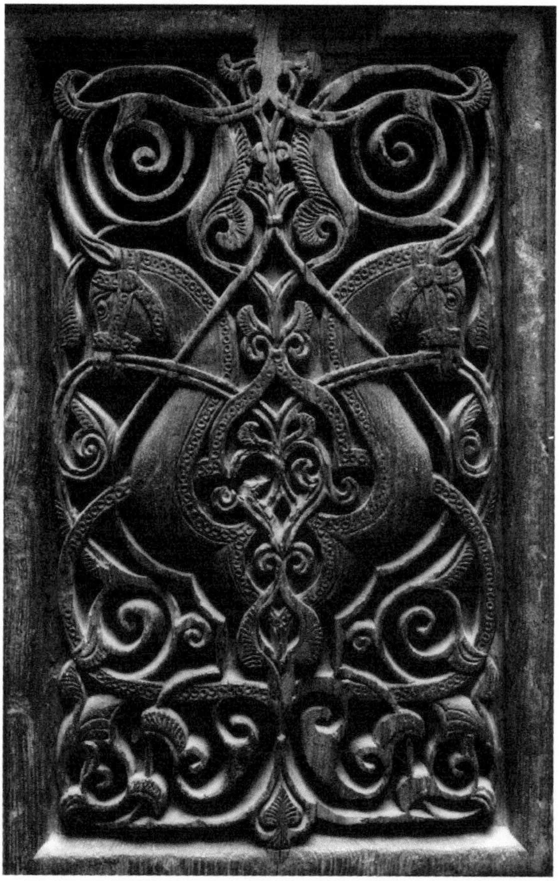

Fatimid wood panel, Cairo, 11th century

> second type is equivalent to the carving, engraving, surface treatment and exteriors of buildings, and the dyes, smoothing, ornaments and fringes on the cloth.[311]

In the Arabian Nights and in Arabic poetry, the beloved woman appears finely dressed and adorned with jewelry. She is admired not only for her natural looks, but for her adornment, which is an integral part of her appearance and the description of it. Ibn al-Ḥājj, a puritanical 14th-century North African scholar, writes in a treatise on Islamic behavior that according to a *ḥadīth*, the equivalent of the *jihād* for women is to please their husbands. He adds that best way to do so is to adorn themselves.[312]

The Prophet is reported to have been hostile to the decoration of mosques and to have said that "the most unprofitable thing that eats up the wealth of a believer is building."[313] All sources agree that the mosque of the Prophet and the early mosques built by his companions were very humble constructions. The sobriety practiced by the early Muslim community is one of the nostalgic themes of orthodox and fundamentalist Islam. In the particular case of architecture, no religious reference or precedent could be used to legitimize its prestige as an art, as happened with music, in whose favor a number of *ḥadīth*s can be quoted, or poetry, which was also recognized despite polemics against the poets. Architecture and its decoration developed a non-dogmatic and non-sacral orientation. Its evaluation, along with that of the other visual arts, was confined to its patrons, the ruling aristocracy, who commissioned the majority of religious and secular monuments and who were also major consumers of artistic products. It thus belonged to the realm of statecraft or *siyāsa*, as a form of political status symbol that was always acknowledged as a necessary part of Muslim politics. The religious establishment did not play a significant role in the patronage of religious institutions; even foundations dedicated to saints and sufis were usually sponsored by the ruling class. Architecture belonged to the realm of politics.

From the viewpoint of ultra-orthodox theologians, any form of embellishment or aesthetic endeavor was suspect as frivolity that could divert the mind away from God. The decoration of mosques, the building of mausoleums, the chanting of the Koran, the melodic call to prayer, music, poetry, figural representations, and in fact any form of artifice that could be interpreted as an expression of vanity, were undesirable. Like the controversy raised in medieval Europe by the Cistercians, in the Muslim world there was a debate between puritans and liberals over the permissibility of ornament in mosques, the use of gold in Koran illuminations, the melodic recitation of the Koran and of the call to prayer (*ādhān*), and the use of music in religious rituals. In the literature dealing with the interpretation of dreams, the stucco decorator represents hypocrisy and falsehood, and the carver, unless he carves Koranic texts, represents vanity, whereas the builder with mud brick carries a positive meaning. The embroiderer, like the jeweler, represents deceit.[314] The history and nature of Islamic art demonstrate, however, that society did not always follow the orthodox path. Majority opinion favored beautifying the Holy Book, and Koran illumination has always been a major art form celebrating its sanctity, and used as a means of facilitating its reading.[315]

The ornamentation of the Koran was not only a matter of illumination. It also functioned in recitation. Just as early Arabic poetry used to be sung, the Koran, when recited, is not simply read, but accompanied by a melody. Several theologians, such as Qurṭubī (d. 1272) and Ibn Qayyim, have explained this phenomenon as part of the ancient Arab passion for music and songs. When the Koran was revealed to them, the Arabs had to dress it in a musical attire. The science of the *qirā'āt*, which is a theological discipline dealing with the modes of reading, vocalization, and pronunciation of the Koran, also includes techniques of melodious recitation. Ibn Qayyim describes the chanting of the Koran as ornamental and refers to a *ḥadīth* of the Prophet recommending the believer to "adorn the Koran with your voices" *(zayyinū al-qur'ān bi-aṣwātikum)*; "everything has its ornament, the Koran's ornament is a beautiful voice" (*inna likulli shay'in ḥilya, wa inna ḥilyat al-qur'ān al-ṣawṭu 'l-ḥasan*).[316] Ultimately, Arab historians and theologians admitted that Koran recitation was closely related to and influenced by the art of music.

The call to prayer is also accompanied by melody, although practice varies from one region to the other, following the attitude of the prevalent legal rite. Since the Ḥanafī rite favors chanting, the most melodious is that performed in Egypt today. In Saudi Arabia, where the Ḥanbalī school of Wahhābī orientation prevails, it is performed very simply and without ornamentation. The first *mu'adhdhin* (man in charge of the call to prayer), Bilāl, was selected by the Prophet for this task on account of his beautiful voice.

The opponents of mosque decoration did not prevail with their argument that ornament diverts the heart (*tashghīl al-qalb*) and seduces the worshiper to neglect prayer, or that the funds allocated for a pious endowment should preferably be spent on the upkeep of the mosque or its enlargement rather than on its ornamentation.[317] Ghazālī, however, condemned the decoration of mosques with the argument that God cares not for silver and gold but only for devoted hearts, supporting his opinion with a Prophet's *ḥadīth* censuring the decoration of mosques and illumination of Koran fascicles.[318] He argued that embellishments in a mosque (*zakhrafa, tazyīn*) divert the worshiper's eyes and heart and may even mislead him to pursue luxury in his daily life (*zakhārif al-dunyā*). Ghazālī's words were mainly addressed to the founders of religious institutions who sought immortality and redemption for their sins by inscribing their names on lavish monuments.

An example of the hostility to embellishment in religious buildings is documented in the chronicle of the Moroccan Ibn Abī Zarʿ. He described the prayer niche (*miḥrāb*) of the Qarāwiyyīn Mosque under the Almoravid dynasty in the 12th century as being encrusted with gold, azure, and other colors so that it dazzled the worshipers to the point of distraction during prayer. When they learned that the Almohads, who were known for their puritanism, were about to conquer their city, the people of Fez started to cover over the decoration of the *miḥrāb* domes with paper and plaster, fearing to be blamed for its lavishness.[319]

The prevailing attitude, however, acknowledged embellishment as a way of venerating and glorifying (*taʿẓīman*) God. The legacy of Arab architecture itself is the strongest evidence that the arguments of austerity could not triumph. Ultimately, the Almohads themselves stopped resisting the seduction of architectural embellishments and used them in their own buildings. In any case, both the opponents and the advocates of architectural embellishment agreed on the principle that aesthetic devices have a significance, either as means of seduction that can divert the heart away from God, or as tokens of piety to be presented to Him. The use of ornament as a form of religious devotion recalls the ancient tradition of donating jewelry to shrines as a token of the donor's devotion.

The significance of architectural ornament as a symbol of the sponsor's piety is even attested in legal documents. Two passages in foundation deeds (*waqf*s) from Mamluk Egypt demonstrate that decorating a mosque and making it pleasing to the eye and to the soul is an act of religious devotion and a generosity to the Muslim community by the sponsor. Foundation deeds are legal documents that include descriptions of the buildings included in the trust and a detailed list of the staff employed in the institution. Although the passages in these *waqf*s are not as subjective as Suger's comments about St. Denis, they deserve our attention, especially since they appear in legal texts.

The first *waqf* is the foundation document for Sultan Qalāwūn's hospital, built in the late 13th century in Cairo. Part of the description of the hospital praises its architecture as outstanding, unparalleled, and famous worldwide for its fine attributes and its beauty (*al-badīʿ bināʾuhu wa 'l-maʿdūm fī 'l-āfāq mithluhu wa 'l-mashhūr fī 'l-aqṭār ḥusnu waṣfihi wa jamāluhu*). The document also praises the perfection that demonstrates its founder's "high aspirations" (*ʿuluww al-himma*).[320]

The foundation deed of Sultan Faraj Ibn Barqūq, written more than a century later (in the late 14th century), is for a religious complex in Cairo.[321] This document is even more emphatic than the first. It includes long passages referring to the aesthetic value of the building interspersed among the usual technical descriptions that form an integral part of the protocol. They refer mainly to the beauty of the decoration. The document describes the mosque as a handsome building, with a pleasing form and agreeable features revealing astounding workmanship. The gilding makes the soul rejoice, the decoration is elegant, outstanding, exquisitely worked, and made of noble, rare, and expensive marbles. Various decorative patterns are described as dazzling, delightful, and rewarding to the eye, rejoicing to the heart and the soul. The fountain is said to quench thirst just by its sight.

Such hyperbole in a legal document cannot be merely ornamental, but must have been intended to convey a message. In the first document, the *waqf* of Qalāwūn, it is said that the beauty of the building demonstrates the founder's high aspirations; in the second it is implied as well. The aesthetic attributes of the monuments are listed together with the items of the estate bequeathed by the sultan for the foundation of his mosque, thus attributing the beauty and excellence of the workmanship to the sultan's efforts. It is his achievement as founder rather than that of the unmentioned craftsmen. This form of displaying piety is exactly what Ghazālī condemned centuries earlier as hypocrisy, when he condemned the decoration of mosques.

The references to the pleasures of the eye, the heart, and the soul leave no doubt that the mosque should have aesthetic features that please God and flatter the worshipers. There is no reference here to any religious symbolism included in the design; it is merely the aesthetic effect that conveys the message of the sponsor's devotion. The preciousness of the material and the virtuosity of the craftsmanship, by pleasing the eye, touch the recipient's heart and soul with happiness. This should attract worshipers to visit the mosque. The political implication is that by sponsoring a handsome public building, the monarch is advertising his own piety. These texts do not, however, convey any idea of the nature of the decorative themes they praise so highly, not even whether they were geometric, floral, or epigraphic.

Ibn Sīnā's statement that Arabic poetry was free of didactic purposes and served only aesthetic needs may also be extended to the visual arts; their significance was to respond to the natural human urge for pursuing pleasure.

The epigraphy of art objects often reveals the high sense of aesthetics that motivated the craftsmen and their clientele. The term beauty is used to express that the purpose of the object was to flatter the beholder. Many objects are compared with a meadow along which the eye wanders. An inscription on a 14th-century mosque in Baghdad tells us that the founder has built, for God's sake and as a token of his devotion, a mosque "delightful and paradisical," as beautiful as an "adorned bride."[322] The entrance to the palace of the Norman king Roger II in Messina had an Arabic inscription that bid the beholder to reverence and contemplate the monument's beauty.[323] Mamluk vessels ask their owners to contemplate their beauty in order to discover all the meanings they include. The foundation inscription of Cairo's Citadel, dated 1183, bearing the name of Ṣalāḥ al-Dīn, states that the building "combines beauty with function." Many inscriptions on North African mosques of various periods allude to the visual beauty of the buildings and their pleasing appearance.

The personification of an art object, whether by letting it speak or by addressing it with speech, was common in the epigraphy of Islamic art. An ivory casket is inscribed with the text *Anā li-'l-ʿayn nuzha* ("I am a delight to the eye").[324] Another one reads:

> The sight I offer is of the fairest, the firm
> breast of a delicate maiden
> Beauty has invested me with splendid raiment
> that makes a display of jewels.
> I am a receptacle for musk, camphor and ambergris.[325]

A similar personification occurs in an inscription on a minaret in Algiers. The minaret praises its own perfection and wonders whether any comparable minaret has ever existed. It eulogizes the efforts of its founder, who made the architecture and the decoration so beautiful that the moon itself, recognizing the beauty of the minaret as equal to its own, paid it homage. The minaret goes on praising its own handsome appearance that lifts the soul and incites admiration, concluding that God has honored the founder who elevated and perfected such a minaret.[326] In the poems inscribed on the walls of the Alhambra the building addresses the viewer, comparing itself to a beautifully dressed bride. Cities and monuments are often compared with *ʿarūs*, which means bride. This simile identifies architectural beauty with feminine attributes combining elegance, adornment, and originality.

Beautiful things in Arabic literature are described in terms of the effect they produce on the beholder. Art is usually said to convey a sense of wonder or marvel at the unique qualities of an object. The term *durra yatīma* (unique pearl), is the current phrase used to convey the sense of incomparably beautiful and valuable. Beauty is qualified as "beyond compare," or "the like of which was never seen."

Unlike the arts in other traditions, Islamic art cannot be interpreted as a form of religious worship or of communicating with the divine, but rather as an aesthetic medium used for displaying pleasing things, artfully produced, either for pleasure or for donation as a pious act. The arts of the Arabs are not metaphoric, not to be understood as revelations of universal wisdom; they were not intended to mean anything other than themselves. It is the context and the user who bestow moral significance upon the work of art. As a profane discipline it obeys only the criteria of the specialists and technicians of each genre and the patron's judgment.

By adopting Aristotle's distinction between the beauty of form and that of content, the Arabs opted for the aesthetic approach. The lack of a systematic visual symbolism, the rarity of human depictions, and a preference for schematic and abstract representations led Islamic art toward a pronounced visuality and aestheticity. Hodgson recognized the significance and the advantage of the aesthetic choice as leading ultimately to the autonomous and eventually secular character of Islamic art which, in a sense, anticipates modernity.[327] Unlike modern art, however, which does not acknowledge any limits to the artist's individuality, Islamic art was limited by a continuity of traditional and formal criteria.

Premodern Muslims had no religious emblem comparable to the Christian cross; the crescent came into use only in modern times.[328] Instead, Koranic verses or the *shahāda* (the first tenet of Islam, stating that there is no God but Allāh and that Muḥammad is His messenger) identified Muslims. Because Muslims received the word of God from God Himself, only the word of God is sacred; all other forms and patterns used in Muslim religious art are interchangeable and multifunctional, and not regarded in themselves as sacred.

The Muslim does not pray in front of any icon or sacral symbol, aside from facing the direction of the Kaʿba in Mecca. This is emphasized by the prayer niche (*miḥrāb*), which centers the Mecca-oriented wall and defines the axis of the mosque. Unlike the cross with its singular character, however, the *miḥrāb* differs little from other decorative niches.

Islamic art is profane in the sense that its characteristic patterns are not regarded as religious symbols; their utilization is neutral and universal. There is no type of ornament that is specifically religious in connotation. Meanings are given by a variety of components, among which the inscription played a major role. The *muqarnas* also had no religious meaning. It was used anywhere, whenever needed. Unlike the stupa in Indian architecture, the Islamic dome was also not a religious symbol, but a structural and aesthetic device used to roof mosques, throne rooms, mausoleums, garden pavilions, *ḥammām*s, ablution fountains, and latrines. In North Africa there are mosques with two domes, one over the *miḥrāb* and the other over the ablution fountain. Function was more decisive in providing the meaning and identifying the buildings than form.

Epigraphy was applied to all objects. Certain Koranic verses were traditionally associated with specific objects or structures because they referred to functions of or associations with these objects: verses about the duty to pray facing Mecca or to give water to the thirsty were found on prayer niches and fountains, respectively; verses referring to death were found on mausoleums. What sometimes appears as symbolic is often merely appropriate on formal grounds. For example, the phrase "in peace and safety enter it (Paradise)" *(udkhulūhā bi-salāmin āminīn,* 15:46), referring to the righteous passing through the gates of paradise, is inscribed indiscriminately on various types of doors and entryways because it includes the notion of entrance. References to the heavens or the firmament were obvious selections to inscribe on domes and ceilings. But there are also many Koranic texts that have a standard application and are found everywhere, such as the Verse of the Throne (2:255), which is acknowledged to be particularly beautiful. There were no strict rules, however. The inscriptions on the minarets of Cairo, for example, show a variety of choices.

The absence of a conceptual and ecclesiastic symbolism in the Islamic visual arts does not imply that symbolism was absent altogether.[329] In dream interpretation, which belonged among the religious sciences, detailed dictionaries were compiled covering all aspects of human life, and including concrete as well as abstract subjects, to indicate their symbolic meaning in dreams. The interpretations are based on associations mainly from the Koran and the *ḥadīth*, but also from written sources and folklore. All kinds of plants, furniture, instruments and utensils were thought to have symbolic meaning. The astonishing fact that these symbols had no particular impact on the visual arts is a strong evidence for the non-purposeful and aesthetic nature of these arts.

Architecture is a universal medium of commemoration; in Islamic cultures as in others, monuments and art objects were created for particular

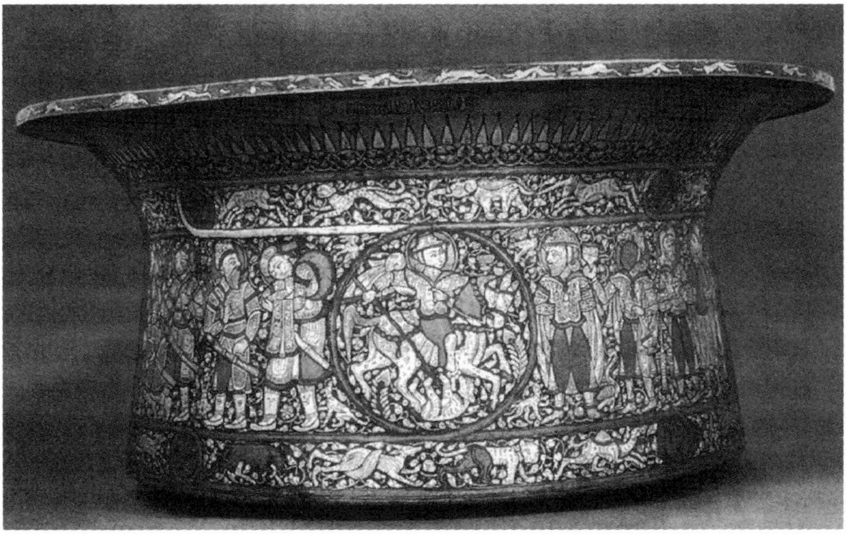

"Baptistère de St. Louis," Egypt, 13th century

events, to celebrate triumphs or commemorate historic moments. The Dome of the Rock (late 7th century C.E.) is the most famous and most discussed example of programmatic architecture, celebrating the triumph of Islam as the third and final monotheistic religion. The metal basin known as the Baptistère de St. Louis is loaded with political reminiscences celebrating al-Ẓāhir Baybar's reforms.[330] The symbolism involved here was not based on a canon or a system of forms and patterns; it was "occasional," not systematic.

Poetry followed pre-Islamic literary ideals, and religious sciences focused on the time of Prophet and his companions, but the visual arts had no particular early models. They evolved through practice, following various sources of inspiration without religious constraint and, as a result, with no opposition between the sacral and profane domains. The first mosques were built according to the plan of the Prophet's house, which thus shaped the classical hypostyle mosque plan, but this style was not dictated by dogma; a mosque could have any shape. The non-dogmatic and non-sacral character of religious architecture is reiterated by the continuous impact of domestic architecture on mosque plans. Not only was the Prophet's house the prototype of the classical hypostyle mosque, but the Iranian four-*īwān*s plan and the Egyptian *qāʿa* were both borrowed from residential architecture for use in mosque architecture.

Some features, such as figural motifs, were rejected because of their pagan or Christian associations; the use of the concave niche as *miḥrāb* was at first controversial because of its association with churches. The Kaʿba, however, in spite of its religious significance in pagan Arabia, became the major shrine under the new religion. In the secular domain, there was no inhibition about using foreign symbols; on the contrary, Muslim monarchs adopted a whole range of symbols of power in their courtly ceremonies and arts. The Arabic "mirror of princes," for example, was a syncretistic genre that took its models from both pre-Islamic and non-Muslim cultures.[331]

The Decorative Themes

IMAGES

Artistic approaches varied across periods and regions. Some regions, such as the Maghreb, hardly made use of figural motifs in their arts from the outset; the arts of other regions, such as Egypt and Syria, became less iconic over time. Western art historians tend to overemphasize the religious motivation behind the non-figural character of Islamic art, for legislation alone does not provide the complete explanation. The prohibition against figural representations is not rooted in the Koran, nor was it always categorical.[332] Although originally shaped by various political, religious, and social factors, taste eventually developed its own criteria. Wine drinking and homosexuality, both far more strictly prohibited by religion than figural representations, were recorded in literary sources as facts of life. Both activities never ceased to be enjoyed and even celebrated in poetry and literature. In the *Arabian Nights* one of the tales deals with a contest between a woman and a man, each advocating the respective advantages of heterosexual and homosexual relationships.[333]

In the early history of Islam under the impact of pre-Islamic Greek, Coptic, and Persian art, mural paintings and sculptures in secular architecture celebrated sporting activities, courtly scenes, and female beauty with figural representations. Even portraiture was occasionally practiced; Omayyad caliphs were represented in paintings and sculptures, and in the 9th century Khumārawayh, the Tulunid ruler of Egypt, had statues of his slave girls made. Portraits of court poets with excerpts of their poems were painted on the walls of Fatimid pavilions, and even the orthodox Mamluk sultan Baybars had his amirs portrayed on the walls of one of his palaces to celebrate his military victories and demonstrate the greatness of his court.[334] Religious buildings and art objects, however, remained aniconic.

After the 14th century, figural depiction disappeared in most of the Arab world, though animal motifs continued for a while to decorate portable objects. Religious strictures alone do not account for this development; a general inclination toward abstract expression characterizes the arts of the Arab world, as confirmed by the abstract treatment of vegetal motifs, which are not prohibited by religious restrictions. Trees and plants were not copied faithfully from nature, but stylized and transformed into unreal linear compositions. The plants in Arabic art can rarely be identified in botanical terms, not because of religious piety, but rather out of a preference for non-realistic and non-narrative artistic expression. Even the disappearance of figural representations was part of a gradual evolution from realism toward stylization. The spirit of late Hellenistic and Christian arts in Syria and Egypt gave way to a more emblematic form of imagery. Musicians and dancers were no longer rendered as feminine as in Omayyad and Fatimid arts, but increasingly as neutral figures of unidentifiable gender, appended to enthroned rulers as symbols of royalty. This evolution reflects the sociopolitical changes in the structure of the ruling establishment.

Although figural representations were far from being a constant or a characteristic element in the arts of the Arab world, Arabic authors have on various occasions discussed the meaning of images. Figural motifs were often understood as having magic or therapeutic powers. Ghuzūlī, a 13th-century scholar, wrote that the *ḥammām* "should contain pictures of high artistic merit and great beauty, representing pairs of lovers, gardens and beds of flowers, fine galloping horses and wild beasts; for pictures such as these are potent in strengthening the powers of the body, whether animal, natural or spiritual."[335] Another medieval author quoted in many books dealing with the advantage of the *ḥammām* wrote:

> All physicians, philosophers and wise men agree that the sight of beautiful pictures gladdens and revitalizes the soul, freeing it from melancholy; it strengthens the heart more than anything because it rids it of all evil thoughts. Some say, if actual beautiful forms are not present, the eyes should turn toward beautiful images produced with excellent workmanship such as pictures in books, monuments, palaces or in baths. All this has been strongly recommended by the philosopher and physician Muḥammad Ibn Zakariyyā al-Rāzī to all who are victims of bad thoughts or evil obsessions that are not in harmony with the order of nature. He said, "When a beautiful picture combines nice colors such as yellow, red, green, and white, with forms of harmonious proportions, it repels the melancholic humors, expels

> the grief that clings to the soul and frees it from sadness, for the mind relaxes and rejoices at the sight of such images and its anxiety is dissipated." He said: "Think of the sages of the past who reflected about the bath over the years, and how they recognized with their sharp and acute mind that one loses a great deal of energy in the bath. With intelligence they found a means to compensate this loss, so they painted three different types of magnificent pictures in beautiful and pleasing colors; these were made to address man's animal, spiritual and natural potentials. They depicted young men fighting, hunting, and horse racing to stimulate the animal potential, they painted scenes with lovers embracing each other, or blaming each other to stimulate the spiritual potential, and they addressed the natural potential with landscapes of gorgeous trees with flowers and radiant colors."[336]

Images, like talismans, can emit the powers characteristic of the objects they represent. The effect of *ḥammām* paintings is further demonstrated, though indirectly, by the following episode. The scholar and litterateur Ibn Ḥazm listened one day to a friend telling him how he fell in love with a woman he saw only in a dream. Ibn Ḥazm was astonished and criticized his friend's folly, saying, "If you had fallen for one of those pictures they paint on the walls of the public baths, I would have found it easier to excuse you."[337]

Because images were believed to have power, they were used for apotropaic purposes and in order to conjure up good fortune. Like the talisman, which deters evil powers, the image can conjure up positive ones. A medical book recommends for specific therapies the use of an amulet with the image of a lion. A ring with a scorpion was believed to deter insects, or the image of a bird depicted on the columns of a mosque in three different places would keep the birds away from the premises.[338] Masʿūdī, speaking of Alexandria, writes that Alexander the Great ordered effigies of maritime demons to be posted along the shores of his city to deter them from harassing the population. When the monsters came out and saw the effigies, they ran away and never came back. Arabic historians, in their long descriptions of ancient Egyptian monuments, point to the talismanic and apotropaic meaning of their inscriptions and icons.

The prominent role of princely imagery among figural motifs is very often to be interpreted in this magic sense. Princely iconography was used not only on objects for princely use, but also on art objects commissioned by the bourgeoisie. Enthroned figures enjoying princely pastimes, such as music and the hunt, prevailed over themes from everyday life. Themes of everyday life, as they were rendered in the *Maqāmāt* of Ḥarīrī, were not popular; princely themes were understood not as mere descriptions of royal pastimes, but rather as allusions to an affluent and successful life similar to that of kings, that had an auspicious meaning for the owner of the art object.[339] They were thus equivalent to the stereotypic epigraphs which usually accompany this imagery and which wish the owner glory, happiness, prosperity, wealth, excellence, victory, authority, power, longevity, and so on. Princely imagery conveyed the message "May you live like a king!" Royalty was a symbol of happiness. The happy ending of a tale is always associated with a kingdom; the merchant marries the king's daughter and becomes king himself.

Similarly, the signs of the zodiac, another major theme of figural representations, were adopted to conjure up an auspicious constellation, as a symbol of good fortune. Votive inscriptions evoking good fortune to the owner, combined with astrological symbols, were characteristic features of objects of practical use such as dishes, bowls, and buckets. The use of princely titles and blazons in the Mamluk period on objects made for persons who did not themselves belong to the aristocracy could also have had an auspicious meaning analogous to that of princely imagery. In the later Mamluk period, when images become rare, we find references to the zodiac inscribed on metalwork showing that words, like images, conjured an auspicious constellation.

As other religions and beliefs associate supernatural powers with images and icons, in Islam such powers are attributed to the Koran. Koranic texts, like the cross in Christianity, are used for apotropaic purposes. In popular religion, specific Koranic verses were, and are, inscribed in amulets against evil or disease. Epigraphy in the arts was often used to this end.

CALLIGRAPHY

As the language of the Koran is inseparable from its divine essence, Arabic and its writing remained the foremost expressions of Muslim identity. Because the Koran represents the direct divine speech, its written word, like its visual expression, came to occupy in Islamic art a place unparalleled in any other culture. "Arabic script is the central form of Islam's arts and was the first and is the foremost of its characteristic modes of visual expression," writes A. Welch.[340] Equivalent in a sense to the icon in Christian culture, calligraphy was valued at all times and places. The genesis of calligraphy was related to the necessity of writing down the Koran, which at the outset was transmitted orally, in a clearly legible form accessible to everyone. In a society that regarded knowledge as of foremost value, literacy was widespread, especially among urban populations, and writing became a major art. As the materialization of God's eternal word, calligraphy is also associated with piety. Some sufis emphasized the connection between writers' souls and their writing, implying that to be a good calligrapher one had to have a pure soul; certain sufi schools attributed occult properties to the Arabic alphabet. In the Arab world, however, calligraphy was less deeply associated with mysticism than it was among Iranians and Turks. Rather, it was cultivated as "the rhetoric of the pen" to serve practical purposes such as chancery, paleography or the adornment of portable objects. Calligraphy was viewed as the reflection of a clear mind: "A beautiful handwriting speaks for the writer, makes his arguments convincing, and enables him to obtain what he wants," commented the governor of Khurasan ʿAbd Allāh Ibn Ṭāhir on a badly written petition.[341] Ibn al-Muqaffaʿ wrote that "the script is adornment for the prince, perfection for the wealthy, and wealth for the poor."[342] In the 15th century Qalqashandī equated the importance of calligraphy for the written word with that of rhetoric for the spoken word.[343] He also refers to *handasat al-khaṭṭ* or the geometry of writing.

The Arabic script and its calligraphy are the most prominent contributions of the Arabs to the arts of Islam. Calligraphy was a discipline with its own precise and strict rules according to which proportionality was mandatory. It was judged by aesthetic criteria, such as proportions and consistency with the style. To meet such criteria, training and an adequate use of tools were necessary. Even on this subject it is possible to quote the Prophet.[344] Ibn al-Haytham said, "A beautiful script is one whose letters have beautiful-looking shapes and are in beautiful composition with one another. . . Perfect beauty in a script comes from the conjunction of shape and position."[345] For Abū Ḥayyān al-Tawḥīdī handwriting is the garden of knowledge, the pen is the chief of wisdom.[346]

The art of calligraphy was not confined to the Koran or to books. Despite its religious association, the origins of the calligraphic art are to be found in the chancery milieu rather than in the religious establishment. All kind of objects were adorned with the written word. The extensive use of inscriptions on objects of daily use reflected the taste of a literate urban society. An important function of inscriptions was political, publicizing statements that advertised the monarch's power. Architecture was the most visible medium to serve this purpose. Many inscriptions in religious and secular architecture refer to the triumphs achieved by the monarchs, either indirectly through the choice of suitable Koranic texts, or through direct statements, sometimes also expressed in verse, as in the Alhambra.

Calligraphy evolved beyond religious and utilitarian purposes to meet aesthetic needs. The aesthetic function of inscription is mentioned by Bīrūnī, who writes that in the art of carving rock crystal the craftsman can conceal defects in the material by decorating or inscribing its surface.[347] Ornamental inscriptions became, along with the arabesque and geometric patterns, an essential element of decoration. The use of inscription in the arts freed the calligrapher's imagination to create ornamental devices. Especially in the case of Kufic writing, which was not ruled by proportional criteria like the cursive *naskhī*, but obeyed the calligrapher's own aesthetics, the letters were transformed into ornament. They were foliated or floriated, twisted and plaited, knotted, intersected, intertwined in endless geometrics, and even animated with figures.

Cursive styles, more recent than the Kufic, evolved in a secular bureaucratic context promoted by viziers. Credit for their invention and refinement was given to calligraphers whose names were singled out and recorded. Among these numerous cursive styles the *naskhī* acquired the greatest popularity; it was perfected in 10th-century Baghdad. Ibn Muqla (d. 940), who was vizier, is credited with being the inventor of this new standard script based on proportionality and following geometric principles. He created a unit of measurement or module for the letters and fixed their basic and their relative form. The letters had to be *mansūb* (well-proportioned), which is also the name of the style he created. The careers of Ibn Muqla and his successor Ibn al-Bawwāb (d. 1021), who was also an illuminator, were not in the religious establishment but in the state bureaucracy.[348] They were both guided by aesthetic criteria.

Because they were designed according to strict rules of proportion, the *naskhī* letters could not be transformed into ornamental elements, as Kufic letters could, so they were combined instead with richly ornamented backgrounds. On art objects and monuments, Kufic and *naskhī* (or its monumental version the *thuluth*) scripts were used together and often combined. Because the first originated in the religious tradition and the other in a secular milieu, they were often associated with different meanings. Whenever both scripts were applied on the same object, the Kufic was used for the Koranic texts and the *naskhī* for the historical inscriptions. To this day Kufic is preferred for conveying traditional Islamic connotations.

The use of the written word as decorative device implied that Allāh's name and His sayings could become "ornaments," and in fact both God's and Muḥammad's names, as well as Koranic verses, were used in the arts in a manner that a modern viewer would regard as obviously decorative. This blend of the sacral with the ornamental indicates that aesthetic devices could be adopted to express religious devotion. The ornamental function of calligraphy is further demonstrated in the occasional use of pseudo-epigraphy, consisting of letters juxtaposed decoratively without meaning, on art objects.

ARABESQUE AND GEOMETRY

Ḥāzim al-Qarṭājannī, in his analysis of the aesthetic experience, wrote that the reflection of stars, lamps, or trees on the calm surface of a body of water is more appealing to the soul than the appearance of the objects themselves. A statue impresses more than the subject it represents because of the startling effect created by the imitation and the manipulation of the real object through artistic work (*ibdāʿ al-ṣanʿa*).[349] Arabic culture has always been aware of the part artistic representation plays in an aesthetic experience; this awareness was expressed explicitly in literary criticism and implicitly in the visual arts. Reality is less impressive than its artistic image; is this not the quintessence of the Islamic visual arts?

In a discourse dealing with ornament in the visual arts, quoted by al-

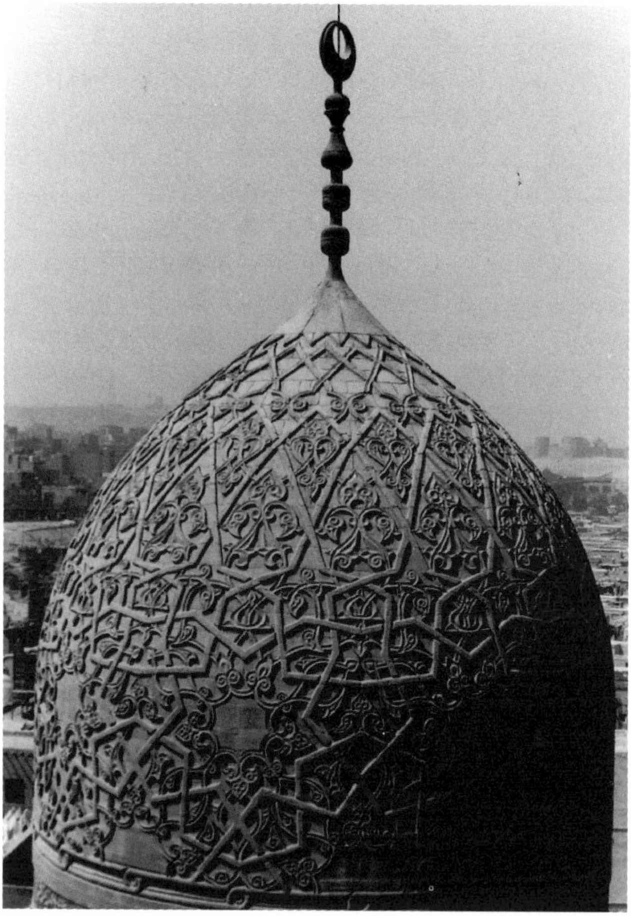

Mausoleum dome of Sultan Qāytbāy, Cairo, late 15th century

Kātib in his book on music, Farābī distinguished between three categories of melodies, the first two of which are of interest here. The first simply produces pleasure; the second and higher stimulates the imaginative faculty of the soul, generating images that recall real things. Farābī compared the first type of melody with ornamental design and the second with figural representations, commenting that ornamental design served to produce pleasure, whereas figural representations expressed human characters and feelings, as did the idols made to personify deities.[350] Farābī's words clearly define non-figural representations as decorative and aimed at stimulating pleasure; he regarded abstract design as aesthetic. Farābī's remarks recall Ibn Sīnā's comparison of Greek and Arabic poetry mentioned earlier. Both philosophers attributed edifying messages to figural and narrative arts and identified non-figural and abstract art with pleasure.

Like Arabic poetry with its preference for far-fetched similes and stylized rather than realistic themes, in the visual arts it is not the individual accidental case that the artist seeks to represent, but the generic principle, the abstract phenomenon. The arts were meant to stimulate imagination rather than narrate facts or episodes. What they seek to convey is not the individual occurrence, but the inward image of it. In his literary criticism, Jurjānī did not follow Aristotle's concept of the arts as mimetic in the sense of imitating reality (*taṣwīr*). Rather, he conceived of poetry and the visual arts as a subjective and creative way of imaginative thinking. Poetry stirs the emotions by establishing similarities between things and thus transforming reality, not by faithfully imitating it, but by generating emotion rather than reporting facts. Abu Deeb, in his discussion of Jurjānī, emphasizes that his comparison of poetry with painting refers to a non-representational, abstract form of art. His concept of "image-making" is not a realistic but a constructional one.[351] Like Ḥāzim al-Qarṭājannī's view of the image as a psychological and not merely visual phenomenon, Jurjānī's view conforms with Ibn al-Haytham's analysis of vision. All three emphasize the psychological depth in the process of artistic perception and the active contribution of the recipient to the artistic experience. It is not the eye alone that is excited, but the intellect as well, as Owen Jones remarked in his analysis of the Alhambra's decoration.

If Muslim orthodoxy stresses that God is the creator of all things and all events, it has never denied or minimized human beings' role in cultivating and fashioning their environment. Because God's absolute power over all things and all events did not allow humankind to act as a creator, the human field of action was focused on elaboration.

As the musicologist al-Faruqi has written,

> Rather than taking nature itself or natural phenomena as his theme—or as his vehicle for expression—and then decorating them with beautifying addendum the Arab artist has made his goal that of expressing himself

> through the manipulation of abstract and stylized motifs. From these he creates compositions conveying a sense of never-ending design. Even if he utilizes figural motifs, they are treated in ways which deny their individuality, their personality or their naturalness. Ornamentation for the Arab artist, therefore, is not an addendum, a superfluous or extractable element in his art. It is the very material from which his infinite patterns are made.[352]

Just as startling poetic images were expected to appeal to the imagination by manipulating the object with similes and poetic language, the arabesque and geometry transcend nature through stylization and abstraction. The same phenomenon is already manifest in the first monuments of Islam. The mosaics of the Dome of the Rock and the Great Mosque in Damascus, in their combination of plants with jewelry and gardens with architecture, reveal the taste for transcended nature. Like the treatment of natural motifs in Arabic poetry and their comparison with jewelry, playful imagination also transcends reality in the visual arts. The tendency to abstraction and stylization, which is already evident in the genesis of the Arab visual arts, is in harmony with the literary tradition that attributed to poetry a higher status than to fiction and narration. Unlike the Iranians, who venerated the *Shāhnāmeh* as history and as poetry and who used it as a major artistic theme in their visual arts, the Arabs separated narration from poetry, which they preferred to enjoy in its abstract form, and their visual arts remained correspondingly less narrative than the Iranian.

The inclination to abstraction and atemporality is present in the Holy Book itself. The Koran, unlike the Old and the New Testaments, narrates neither the history of a people nor the lives of various individuals, though it does tells various stories. As the eternal and sacred word of God, it does not have to be written in chronological order. The *sūras* are arranged by length beginning with the longest. Since the longer ones were those revealed to the Prophet at a later date, the order is even antichronological. The first *sūra,* the *fātiḥa* or overture, is the only exception to this rule. Agglutination rather than methodical narration is the principle here.

One of the characteristic features of Islamic ornament is its preference for organizing a surface rather than singling out a pattern. Pattern and background are not always identifiable or separable. At the same time nothing is unframed or left in its own contours. The frame plays a major

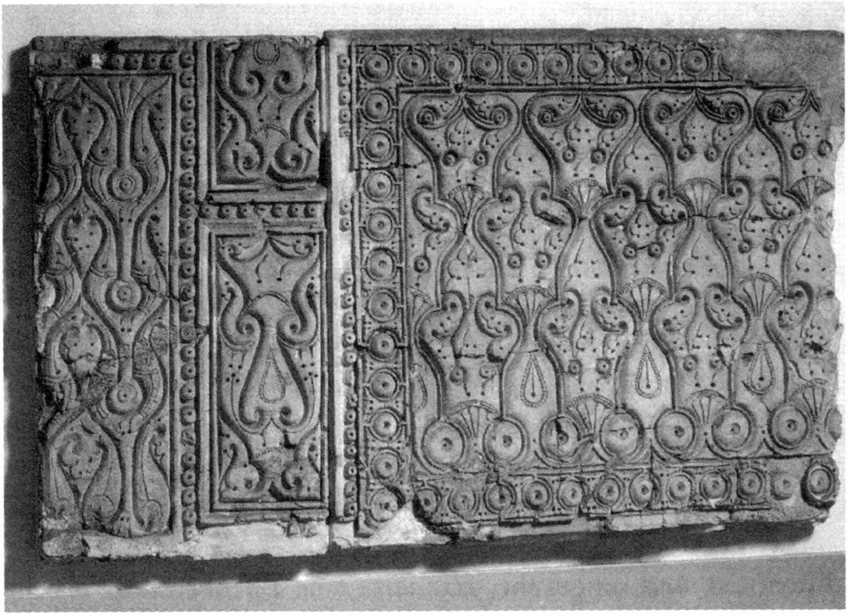

Wall decoration, Samarra, 9th century.

role; whether in architecture or on portable objects, it precedes the content, which is subordinated to it. Inscriptions, arabesques, and geometrics are integrated into a given precalculated surface. Figural motifs are rarely autonomous or monumental; rather, they are included within bands, cartouches, or roundels, alternating with purely ornamental patterns. In pottery, it is the circular shape of the dish that determines the profile of the motif painted on it. There is a preference for juxtaposition rather than hierarchy of themes, a feature to be found in poetry and music as well.

The arabesque was the primary feature that struck Europeans in Islamic art, hence the Western term, which has no equivalent in the Arabic language, to designate floral patterns stylized to abstraction and "geometricized." Western historians and Orientalists also frequently use the term to refer to the non-visual arts in Islam, especially in poetry. Whereas some interpreted the arabesque as an expression of *horror vacui*, Kühnel saw it as aesthetic asceticism.[353] "Intricate" is one of the terms most widely used by art historians to describe Islamic designs.

In the artistic explosion of the Abbasid period, and more particularly in the so-called Samarra style C, lies the origin of the arabesque, which is characterized by the repetition of curved lines without identifiable foreground or background, producing abstract motifs with an ornamental effect. Lines play the major role in this style. No matter what the origins of its patterns, the Samarra style suited the Arabic taste for ambiguity, esprit, and variations on a theme. Like word plays, the relationship and interplay between lines created an image where subject and background were interchangeable according to the viewer's choice. This absence of thematic hierarchy also occurs in poetic similes; the female bosom was often compared with ivory, and vice-versa, an ivory casket also recalled a women's breasts.[354] The poets compare a meadow to brocade and brocade to a meadow.

Arab artists have stylized other motifs besides plants, such as the shell, inherited from classical art, or the sun motif, which they blended with the geometrical star. Stylization consisted basically in giving these patterns a geometric interpretation, in transforming the real into the unreal. The arabesque and Islamic geometrics are closely related. The first consists of an interlace of curved lines representing stylized vegetal motifs forming polygonal figures. The latter consists of interlaced straight lines forming endless star patterns based on either the six- or the eight-pointed star and their derivatives. Geometric designs are often filled or combined with arabesques, in a playful contrast of straight and curved lines, often accentuated with colors.

The interlacing of strands in geometrical designs in complex star configurations conveys an illusion of never-ending movement or rotation. The role of movement in Islamic design has not been emphasized enough. The multifaceted *muqarnas* reflects the movement of light. The *muqarnas* dome at the Hall of the Two Sisters in the Alhambra bears an inscription that refers to the colors revolving in the alternating light between night and day. Ancient myths of rotating domes were known to the Arabs; they are mentioned in association with Greece, ancient Iran, and Egypt. In his history of ancient Egypt Maqrīzī describes a glass dome decorated with astronomical motifs, which rotated following the movement of the planets. Other domes were connected with light towers; a dome surmounting a tower changed its color every day of the week, returning to the first color on the eighth day.[355]

Epigraphy produces movement on the inscribed surface, which the reading eye follows. The movement created by the inscription is framed by a ribbon, one of the most consistent elements on Islamic architecture and portable objects, which is not static but composed of an upper and a lower strand that run parallel and intersect at regular points. In Koran illuminations and metalwork the ribbon appears in a relentless alternation between parallels and intersections in an endless movement encircling the entire page or the vessel, creating a dynamic composition. In Koran illuminations, the same strings that constitute the central geometrical star composition shoot out of the star and turn around it to form the frame. The geometrical star is based on the movement of upper and lower strands, interacting as in basketwork, giving the flat surface a multi-level appearance. Owen Jones in his analysis of Arab ornament noticed that arabesques and geometrical stars are designed on two or three levels, and that the straps or twigs interlock across these levels.

In a geometrical or floral composition, the patterns are not repeated with juxtaposed individual stars or arabesques, but connected as in a net or a canvas in continuity rather than juxtaposition. The most intricate patterns can be traced down to a few strands or branches that interlock and interlace over the entire design. The endless interlace captures and dazzles the beholder. "To dazzle" is a term often used in inscriptions and literature to characterize artistic beauty, both in the positive sense and with negative implications.

This phenomenon of intersection is manifest even in architecture. In western Islamic mosques one arch form is used for the arcades running parallel to the main wall and another for the perpendicular ones. The intersection bays have a third, more elaborate, arch form that accentuates the crossing of the two others, a device that creates an effect of movement.

Thanks to its sense of geometry, Islamic art, with all its exuberance and lavishness, never becomes incoherent or chaotic. Geometry adds a systematic intellectual dimension to art. Its use is pervasive: it rules calligraphy, subjugates floral motifs into methodic geometrical compositions of linear patterns, and sections vaults into *muqarnas*.

In the Arab world, however, geometrical design inspired the builder less than the decorator. Arab mosques are less defined by a geometrical mind than Gothic cathedrals, and they are less symmetrical than the Iranian and Ottoman. In spite of its axiality the hypostyle mosque was open-ended, flexible, and agglutinating. Like the Prophet's mosque, it was not a symmetrical building, but built around a courtyard on the four sides of which rooms and halls of various size and shape were grouped.

To move within the rules of geometry and play with them was a great challenge to artists. Their skill consisted of mastering these rules and operating within them. In geometrical patterns, each line follows a pre-calculated logical path according to rules that have to be mastered through expertise. This kind of design cannot be improvised or produced at random, but it has to be conceived according to a rational concept. In a society that honors tradition and consensus and values science and intellectual dexterity, the rules of geometry embody discipline and convention. They were a form of universal reference or guideline that cannot err. De Bruyne's remark on medieval European art—that it was commanded by know-how, which itself was defined by exact rules, and that the work of art was valued as a masterpiece (*opus subtiliter factum*) if its creation conformed to the technical norms[356]—can be applied to the Arab concept of art as well.

Architecture and Decoration

Ever since the Dome of the Rock was built in the late seventh and the Great Mosque of Damascus in the early eighth century C.E., the arch has been the pivot of Islamic architecture and a fundamental element in its decoration. The hypostyle mosque plan derived from the Prophet's mosque, a simple structure built with palm trunks. The columns were very soon coupled with arches to build arcades. The arch defined not only the structural interior of the mosque, but aesthetic devices as well. It determined the *miḥrāb* as well as windows, niches, and panels, not to mention the *muqarnas*, which is a three-dimensional geometric multiplication of an arched surface. The arch motif was also used on portable objects. It is characteristic of Islamic aesthetics to fuse structural with ornamental devices. At the Great Mosque of Cordova the superimposed arches, which had earlier been used by the Romans in their Iberian aqueducts, are not only structural but integrated into the decorative program, blurring the line between function and aesthetic play. Conversely, the *muqarnas* arches, which are devoid of structural function, often appear as if they were supports.

Domestic architecture shared the decorative devices displayed in sacral buildings; the architectural forms, however, remained faithful to local traditions. Exterior decoration was rare and luxury was confined to the interior, reflecting the Islamic attitude toward the privacy of domestic life.

It is a mistake to speak, as has often been done, of *horror vacui* as a principle of Islamic art. As has been brilliantly demonstrated by Marçais, ornament was not applied like wallpaper on buildings, but was subordinated to the architectural design.[357] Decoration was applied not haphazardly, but to accentuate the architectural elements and structural compositions, interacting with them either by disguising or by revealing them. Patterns were categorized according to the nature and form of the decorated surface. *Muqarnas*, for example, was not applied to flat surfaces. Inscriptions were shaped in horizontal bands.

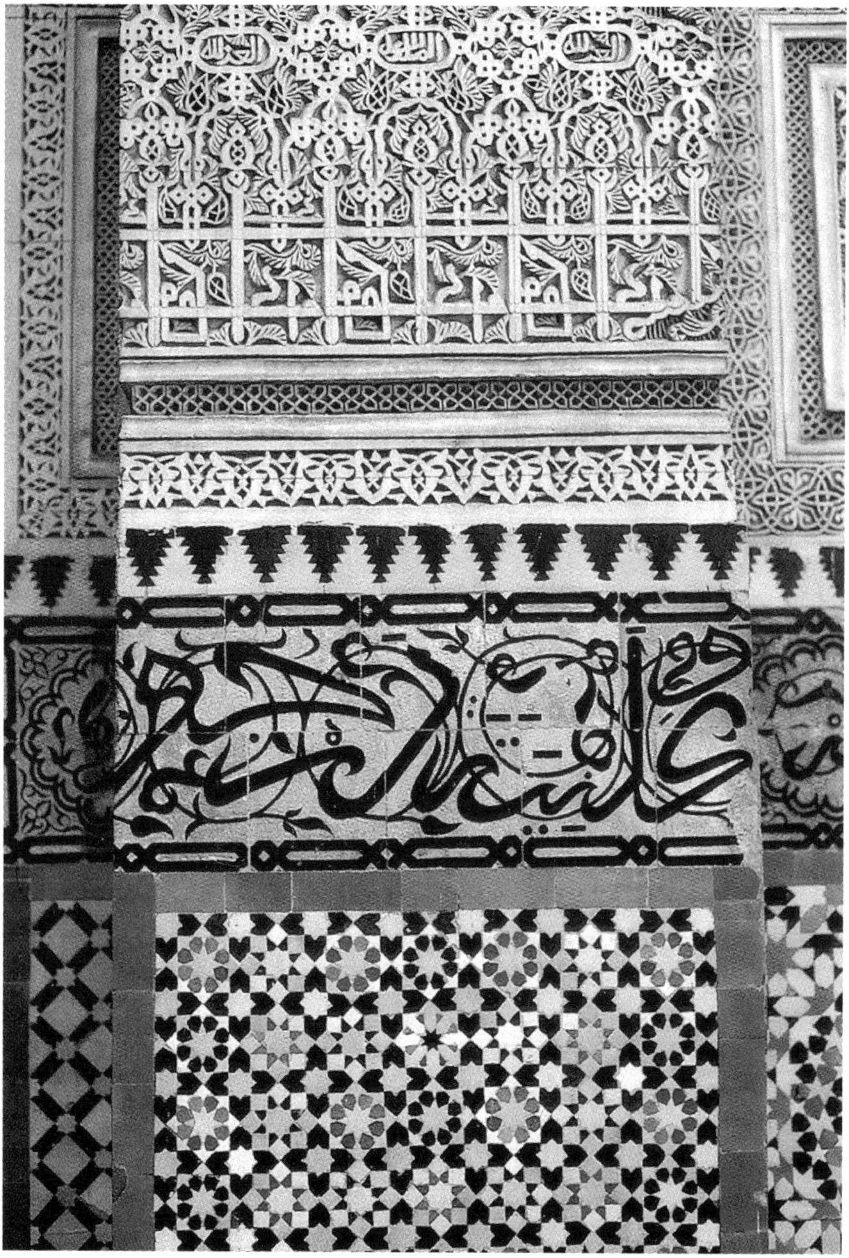

Wall decoration in the *madrasa* of Abū ʿInān in Meknes, 14th c.

There are two main principles, a liturgical and a formal one, in the disposition of ornament in a mosque. The first takes into account the necessity of praying toward the Kaʿba, and thus of giving the mosque a corresponding orientation. The *miḥrāb* is not a necessity, however, for finding the Mecca orientation, since the sanctuary itself is built along a Mecca-oriented axis and the worshiper need only face the main wall. The *miḥrāb* is the place where the *imām*, who conducts the prayer, stands. At the outset the prayer leader was the Prophet, then the caliph, and finally any learned man from the community. Since the prayer niche is on the main axis of the mosque, the accentuation of this area also has a formal geometrical aspect; with time it acquired an autonomous aesthetic function. In all mosques from all periods, the most decorated part of the interior is the *miḥrāb* and the area around it. It was emphasized first ornamentally and later also architecturally, with the superimposition of a cupola and the creation of a transept or a wider central aisle. Ways of enhancing the *miḥrāb* vary according to period and place; even the absence of ornament may be a means of enhancing the *miḥrāb* area. In Moroccan and Tunisian mosques and *madrasa*s, the polychrome ceramic dadoes, characteristic of the courtyard of the building, were not used inside the prayer hall, where the *miḥrāb* was decorated only with stucco. In residential architecture, as in the Alhambra, there was no restraint in the use of interior decoration except in the oratories, which lack the ceramic decoration. In Mamluk funerary complexes the mausoleum was often more decorated than the mosque, indicating a certain reluctance about decorating sanctuaries.

The occasional visual parallel between portal and *miḥrāb* is merely formal, not symbolic, a result of both being regarded as main elements to be highlighted in a religious building. Both structures are arched, because the use of the arch and its decorative repertoire was universal.

The second principle in architectural decoration was the accentuation of architectural elements such as arches, openings, and transitional zones. The arches dictated the general decorative design. Once the basic lines of the arches with their frames, voussoirs, and spandrels were drawn, the intermediate spaces were subsequently treated with vertical or horizontal designs according to their configurations. Each section of the arch, voussoir, soffit, or spandrel had a specific pattern. At the Dome of the Rock, the palm trees and vases made of glass mosaic are subordinated to the shape of the surface they adorn. Applied on a rectangular pier, the trees acquire a rectangular silhouette. The soffits are filled with repetitive patterns and the spandrels with corresponding triangular scroll compositions. The inscription band follows the junction between the wall and the ceiling.

Ornament did not conceal the framework; rather it emphasized connections between vertical and horizontal elements, articulated links and joints, and framed accesses and openings. *Muqarnas* may be applied to conceal a pendentive or transform a vault, but its sheer presence and placement signal a sensitive point. Craftsmen all over the Muslim world have given the transitional zones of the domes the greatest artistic attention as the most sensitive and critical parts of a domed structure. Even where ornamentation was heavily applied, such as the Dome of the Rock, the Alhambra, the Madrasat al-ʿAṭṭārīn in Fez, or the funerary mosque of Qāytbāy in Cairo, it was applied not uniformly, but in relation to architectural structure.

On the exteriors of mosques, the most prominent elements were the gateway and the minaret. Both structures signal the presence of the mosque, the minaret at a distance and the gate from closer up. As in most architectural traditions, the gateways of Islamic monuments were articulated with decoration, and later with architectural devices such as a monumental portal or a minaret above the entrance. The gate both leads the believer into the mosque and marks the axis of the building. According to Marçais, the entrance is the magnificent preface to the sanctuary, equivalent to the frontispiece of a book, which, as in Koran fascicles, is the most densely illuminated page.

Inscriptions were rarely applied in vertical panels, but rather in horizontal bands running around the building, highlighting and framing walls and their openings. Inscription bands often mark, like a belt, the junction between two distinctive sections, such as the dado and the upper wall. As horizontal elements they were used to adorn the drums of domes, both inside and out. In a decorative program otherwise defined by arches, niches, and panels, inscribed bands were the main horizontal element and thus had a counterbalancing and integrating effect.

After the creation of the Samarra style of decoration, building craftsmen achieved a high degree of standardization in their working methods.

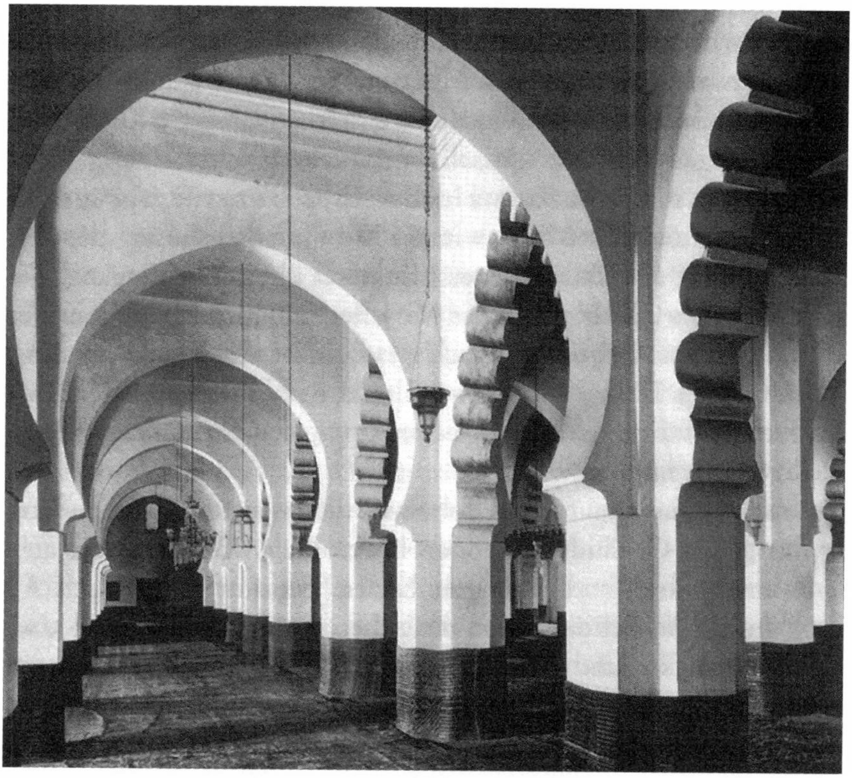

Great Mosque of Algiers, 11th century

Ceilings, dadoes, pavements, domes, minarets, and arches had their respective decorative designs. Once the broad architectural lines were set, the rest could be left to the highly specialized craftsmen operating with preconceived modules. The open-ended and agglutinating character of geometrics and arabesques facilitated standardization. Although the *muqarnas* is not agglutinating, but mostly conceived around a focal point, standardization characterized *muqarnas* vaults as well; with only a small number of elements—at the Alhambra there are only seven—endless combinations could be generated.

In contrast with Ottoman, Timurid, and Safavid religious architecture, monumentality is not a characteristic feature of mosques in the medieval Arab world. This seems to be a matter of evolution. In the great mosques of the classical age from North Africa to India, horizontality rather than verticality prevailed. Only the minaret conveyed verticality. The period of monumentality was post-medieval; at that time most of the Arab regions were provinces of Ottoman Empire. But even in the golden ages of the Hafsids in Tunis, the Merinids in Morocco, and the Mamluks in Egypt and Syria, monuments were not designed to be bold and massive. The uncompleted monumental mosque of Sultan Ḥasan in Cairo was an exception. The goal of the Mamluks had been rather to adorn their cities, especially their capital Cairo, with a dense net of handsome monuments. Their architecture was to be omnipresent rather than central and dominant.

Buildings were originally more colorful than they appear today. Woodwork (especially the ceilings), stucco, and marble were painted with red, lapis lazuli blue, and green, with an abundance of gold, particularly in epigraphy. Colored glass filled the pierced stucco window panels. Polychromy was most accentuated at the level of the dadoes, whether with marble or ceramic decoration, contrasting with the more subdued upper wall. But the taste for cladding architecture with decoration did not pervade all of Islamic architecture. Unlike those of later Iranian and Central Asian architecture, the aesthetics of the Mediterranean Muslim world did not favor entirely wrapping the exterior of buildings with a mantel of colored ornaments or glazed tiles. Preference was given rather to setting accents and operating with contrasts. This was done by carving, gilding or covering domes or minaret tops with glazed tiles to contrast with the plain walls, or by using striped two-colored masonry on certain parts of the building.

Unity, Diversity, and Transmission of Knowledge

Orientalists of the past linked the arabesque with the *Weltanschauung* of the Muslim peoples and the *muqarnas* with the character of Islam, a cultural classification that no longer appeals to contemporary scholarship, which views the arts of Islam in a more autonomous way. It is ornament, however, that most characterizes Islamic art to the non-Muslim beholder. Modern art historians like to speak of the dichotomy in Islamic art between regionalism and universality, pointing to the presence, on the one hand, of typical and characteristic Islamic features, often identified as expressing the unity of Islam, and, on the other, to regional particularities that counteract stylistic homogeneity.

This duality between regional and universal features in Islamic art is not random. There seems to be a certain regularity in this phenomenon, which is related to technology and its transmission. The art of surface treatment was universal; calligraphy, arabesques, geometrics, and *muqarnas* characterized traditional Islamic art. Not only were ornamental patterns ubiquitous; so was the system of their disposition on the ornamented surface. Not just the *muqarnas* and the inscription band, but the association of the *muqarnas* with vaults and transitional zones, and the use of inscription bands to frame portal gates and prayer niches, were found everywhere. Regionalism became increasingly evident in techniques and architectural forms over time.

The diffusion of Islamic ornamental devices on the one hand, and the regionalism of architectural forms on the other, indicate that linear designs were easier to transmit than architectural technology. The *muqarnas,* although universal as a decorative principle, was technically attuned to regional building methods. Similarly, ceramic wall revetment, which was applied in the Maghreb as well as in Central Asia, with geometrical, calligraphic, and arabesque patterns, was executed in each region with different techniques. The arch was used universally, though each region had its own form and its own technique of centering.

The universal features belonged not to the technological but rather to the conceptual and ornamental aspects of architecture, which could be communicated with words, or transmitted with drawings or portable objects, without large-scale migration of craftsmen.

Under normal circumstances transferring architectural knowledge could not have been easy. Muslim building craftsmen traveled less frequently than their European counterparts and their countrymen from the scholarly establishment because of the nature of the political and economic systems of the Muslim world. The rulers monopolized the building trades, their sheer importance as employers having a decisive impact on them. They were the sponsors of most of the religious, military, and commercial buildings, and they alone carried out all infrastructural and military projects. This centralization of the building trades discouraged migration of craftsmen on a large scale, for example as workshops. Unlike their European counterparts, medieval Arab craftsmen did not manage to form autonomous corporations or guilds to speak for their own professional interests. The rulers could summon or dispatch craftsmen, and in times of war they deported them as booty. Large-scale migrations of craftsmen occurred only in periods of catastrophe, as in the case of the Mongol invasions or the Spanish Reconquista.

The regionalism of architecture in the traditional Muslim world was also a side effect of the absence of architecture as an academic discipline like medicine or music. Had it been taught on a theoretical basis, it would have acquired a universal character like other disciplines, and would have been transmitted through books or through the ulema. There was no limit to the transfer of the literature on law, medicine, or mathematics from the Maghreb to India. Cordovan medical books were used and translated centuries later by Ottoman physicians; legal treatises from Samarqand were applied in Cairo. Abbasid mathematical manuals were used and translated by the Timurids in Central Asia. Architecture, however, was essentially an empirical technique. Innovations resulted from experimental and tentative work rather than artistic fervor or ad-hoc creations; architectural breakthroughs were reached cautiously, working from empirical knowledge rather than bold design. They were thus cumulative and collective rather than individual achievements.

Architectural innovations were also motivated by functional adjustments. One of the major innovations in Islamic architecture was the adoption of the four-*īwān* plan in mosque architecture to partly replace the traditional hypostyle hall. The reason was the creation of the *madrasa*, a boarding religious institution, which needed living units for its students and therefore required a layout different from that of the classical mosque. Gradually the lines between the *madrasa* and mosque were blurred and the *madrasa* plan was assimilated into mosque architecture. In any case it was not the invention of an individual artist.

Religious or intellectual movements played no role in artistic evolution, unlike geopolitical factors. Omayyad art acquired its main features from the fact that Damascus, with its Byzantine tradition, was the imperial capital, and Abbasid art was marked by Irano-Mesopotamian culture arising from its geographical and political affinities with Baghdad. The emergence of the Samarra style coincided with the foundation of that new capital city by the Abbasid caliphs.

When foreign architectural forms were adopted, only the basic idea or design was transferred, whereas the practical application, which included the proportions, was adapted to local technology. The mosque of Ibn Ṭūlūn in Cairo was inspired by the architecture and decoration of imperial Samarran mosques; its spiral minaret, however, unlike its prototype, was made of stone instead of brick, and with a rectangular rather than circular base. The idea of making a spiral exterior staircase, but not the technique, came from Samarra. This general idea was easy to transmit—it could be done by oral communication—but the details of the elevation needed communications more complex and accurate than oral transmission could convey. Historians report an apocryphal story according to which Ibn Ṭūlūn was playing with a piece of parchment, turned it around his finger, and thereupon conceived the idea of building his minaret in a spiral shape. This episode demonstrates that design could be transmitted by gesture. The minarets at the mosque of al-Nāṣir Muḥammad in the Citadel of Cairo are adaptations in stone of an Iranian brick prototype. The difference that results affects not only material and proportions but ultimately the whole character of the structure. The four-*īwān*s plan in a Cairene *madrasa* has only the idea in common with Iranian mosques; all other architectural features are determined by local building technology.

Ottoman-style mosques erected in Egypt and Iraq show a similar combination of imported plan and local building methods.

In the case of portable objects, replication was naturally easier to manage. The famous Pisa griffon, a bronze sculpture, has been variously attributed by art historians to Iran, Egypt, and Spain. The original can often be identified by the inscription. Islamic ornament, which is based on linear patterns, did not depend on the migration of craftsmen for its transmission, since it could be transmitted by portable objects or on paper, explaining its universal application in many materials and a variety of objects. The same patterns used in Koranic illuminations appear on vessels and in architectural decoration. Koran illuminators seem to have played an avant-garde role in the spread of ornamental devices. There is almost no pattern used in Koran illuminations that does not turn up in other arts, such as architecture and most particularly metalwork. This commonality should not be directly linked to the sacred meaning of the Koran, however, and interpreted in religious terms. Rather, the Koran's sacred significance required that patrons assign the most prominent designers and painters to create designs for it, which then became widespread. Once the design was on paper, its diffusion across geographical borders and its application in a variety of materials and techniques was easy. The spread of chinoiserie in medieval Islamic arts, including architectural decoration, occurred as a result of the China trade; its patterns were diffused by portable objects such as porcelain and textiles. The yearly pilgrimage to Mecca provided a great opportunity for all kinds of exchange and interaction between Muslims from all over the world, from China to Morocco. Islamic urban society was literate and mercantile. What could be transmitted on a portable object was easily copied. The techniques and the modes of application of the patterns, however, which were the domain of the craftsmen, remained a matter of local tradition.

Construction techniques were mainly learned through apprenticeship rather than taught as a science based on theory; the transmission of architectural expertise would have been practicable only through itinerant workshops, which do not seem to have been common. What gave Islamic art its overall character were its ornamental principles.

Regalia and Luxury

For Ibn Khaldūn, all activities in the sciences, arts, crafts, and trades could flourish only in a city and with princely patronage. Their progress cannot be detached from urban culture because they depend on economic activity and growth, which produce affluence, which in turn generates demand for luxury goods. This demand stimulates the rulers to sponsor arts and sciences, thus displaying their wealth and manifesting their power. Palaces, gardens, elegant furniture, luxurious vessels and garments are the products of affluence and princely patronage. Ibn Khaldūn identifies the arts as the symbols of wealth and power. Because affluence is necessary to produce arts and crafts, the display of refinement is an expression of political power. Luxury and extreme refinement, however, also bear the seeds of decline and decadence. Ibn Khaldūn, who was the first to interpret history in terms of cycles with beginning, apogee, and downfall comparable to the biological life cycles, regarded the culmination of a historical phase as marking the beginning of its decline. An excess of opulence and comfort softens the people, they lose vigor and zeal and become increasingly unmanly.[358]

A major manifestation of Islamic art was the production of luxury objects for the rulers and the bourgeoisie. Luxury in the courtly context meant power; for the urban bourgeoisie it served pleasure and represented social prestige. The most detailed descriptions of art objects that can be found in Arabic literature deal with royal regalia. In spite of the hostility of orthodox theologians against the frivolity implied in the use of luxury and their disapproval of decorating palaces with gold that could otherwise have been invested in the holy war, historians in general tended to favor rulers who cultivated traditional ceremony and to criticize those who neglected it. Sumptuous courts belonged to the monarch's image, as a venue for ceremonies and parades and a medium for displaying the grandeur of Islam to the non-Muslim world. Even the most orthodox minds acknowledged that for the reception of Christian ambassadors,

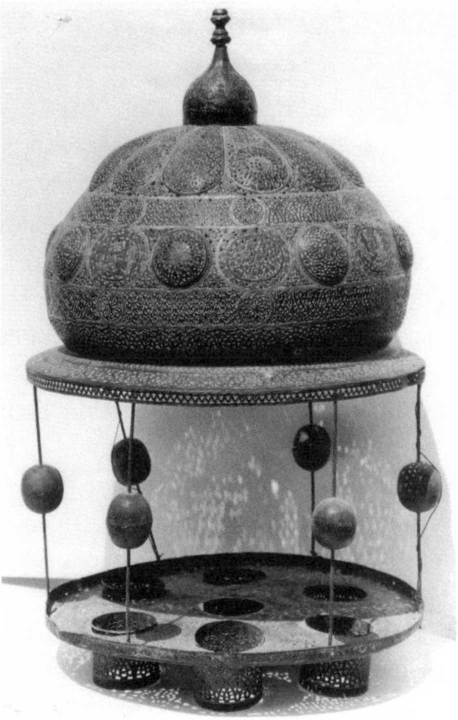

Mamluk metal lamp, Egypt or Syria, 15th century

the monarch should display all possible grandeur to impress the visitor with the glory of Islam; all that served Muslim interests was permissible, and the display of art and luxury served the glory of Islam.[359] Indeed, the Christian world's image of Arab culture was one of luxury and sensuality. It overwhelmed Westerners from the Crusaders in the 11th century to artists in their encounter with the Orient in the 19th century. In 1096, while the Byzantine emperor Alexius Comnenus awaited the onslaught of the Crusaders on his territory, hordes of locusts swept over the country, leaving the grain untouched but destroying the vine. Soothsayers, with wishful thinking, said this meant the Crusaders would spare the Christians, symbolized by the grain which is the source of bread and life, but would destroy the Arabs, whose sensuality was symbolized by the vine.[360]

The royal palaces had collections or treasuries of art objects, which on special occasions were shown off to official visitors. But sheer pleasure in beautiful things was involved as well. An Arabic literary genre specialized in the description of treasures and rarities collected by kings (*al-tuḥaf wa 'l-dhakhā'ir*), including the gifts they received and those they offered. Besides gems, the collections included objects cherished for their extraordinary character, such as statuettes of excellent craftsmanship and striking realism made of precious material. The artistic beauty required to serve the representative functions of the monarchs and to entertain them was accomplished when the virtuosity of the craftsman coupled with the preciousness of the material resulted in a unique object. Landscapes and animals made of gold and silver encrusted with precious stones, a golden peacock with eyes of rubies and feathers of enameled glass and golden threads, a cock made of gold with a ruby comb encrusted with precious stones, or a garden with fruit trees made of silver and gold combined with other precious materials, like later creations of Italian Renaissance artists, generated great excitement at the court and were described in unusual detail by historians.[361] But Islamic artists also attained a refined level of workmanship on cheap material. Very few silver and gold objects have survived, but pottery and metalware demonstrate that common materials were manufactured to highly sophisticated standards.

Exotic and unusual objects, such as gifts from India or China, were admired and greeted with enthusiasm, even if they had pagan associations. A brass idol, probably from India, representing a bejeweled woman with four arms seated in a wagon drawn by dromedaries, was sent from a Khurasanian governor to the caliph in Baghdad, where it made a great sensation. The people nicknamed the idol *shughl*, "a hard day's work" because everyone left his work to go and see it while it was on display.[362] The arrival of a gorgeous tent at the court of the Mamluk sultan al-Ghūrī was similarly celebrated with curiosity and fun. It had originally belonged to a king of Iraq, from whom it was captured and brought to Persia. The Persian Shah Ismāʿīl sent it as a gift to Sultan al-Ghūrī, who ordered it to be put on display. The chronicler Ibn Iyās describes it in unusual detail as circular, lined with blue felt and with red silk ropes. The wood was painted with decorations of trees, birds, and fighting animals. The floor was covered with a round carpet of rare designs.[363] The value of an art object manifested the owner's importance, no matter how he acquired it, whether by order, by purchase, as booty, or as a gift.

Throughout the Middle Ages the Muslim world was a supplier of luxurious textiles and it was a substantial importer as well. Textiles are mentioned in all descriptions of princely treasures, booty and dowries. Arab chroniclers listed the royal wardrobe and textile collections and the royal tents as belonging among the royal regalia. Robes of honor were the greatest signs of distinction that could be bestowed upon a subject.

Appointment to a high position in state was celebrated with the bestowal of a corresponding robe. Furniture and draperies were valued and iconographic textiles had a significant place in courtly arts.[364] Textiles were analogous to murals, with the advantage that they could be replaced to suit the occasion. Curtains fulfilled ceremonial functions by concealing and revealing the caliph as in a theater. Some royal textiles were designed to express political power. The mantle of the Norman king of Sicily, Roger II, made by Arab craftsmen and inscribed with Arabic inscriptions, shows the allegoric image of a feline attacking a camel underneath a palm tree, probably a symbol of Christian triumph over Islam.[365] Textiles were inscribed with princely names and titles as well as with poetry. The art of carpet-weaving flourished not only among Iranians and Turks but also in Arab territories.

The holiest Muslim sanctuary, the Kaʿba, is covered with a cloth embroidered with Koranic inscriptions, which is replaced yearly on the occasion of the pilgrimage. The task of covering the Kaʿba as a symbol of religious devotion holds great prestige. Muslim rulers competed and fought for the honor of donating this curtain.

To dress finely and have a beautiful appearance is also a form of reverence to God, as long as it does not lead to vanity. The Koran says "dress well when you attend your mosques" (7:30).

Perfume belonged with elegant attire. The Prophet perfumed himself. In the *Arabian Nights* a visit to the *ḥammām* is completed by wearing new clothes and using perfume. The mosques were perfumed with incense before prayer time and rooms were scented with incense and perfumed candles.

Literary sources tell about fashions created by prominent men and women. Zubayda, the wife of Hārūn al-Rashīd, celebrated in Arabic historiography for her great infrastructural works on the pilgrimage road, was also famous for the fashions she introduced in clothes, head-dress, and furnishings. The 9th-century musician Ziryāb acquired great fame for his influence on the styles of clothes, cuisine, and pastimes at the Omayyad court of Spain.

Islamic art, in spite of its pronounced princely component, was not exclusively aristocratic. The styles and fashions created and sponsored by the aristocracy were adopted by the urban bourgeoisie, who had a significant share as commissioners and consumers of objets d'art. "Islamic art is characterized by aesthetic democratization," wrote Grabar,[366] who points to the significance of the art of the object as an expression of the affluence of a cultivated urban society with an egalitarian disposition. The Muslim urban population approached aesthetics as modern society approaches design, through all aspects of daily life. A historian of Islamic art has to deal not only with palaces and mosques, but with pots and candlesticks as well. Attention was lavished on objects for daily use, which were valued enough to be inscribed with Koranic texts, poetry, homilies, and princely names.

Except for pre-Islamic poetry, which praises desert life and which is still much admired by educated Arabs, the art of the Arabs was essentially urban. Arabic literature is full of passages belittling the peasant and the bedouin, who were not considered to be good Muslims because proper religious practice was possible only in the city, where all institutions of learning and worship were concentrated. This idea is supported by the *Sharīʿa*, which allows Friday mosques only in urban agglomerations where there is a *qadi* and a representative of governmental authority. It was therefore in the cities that Muslim rulers concentrated their patronage and their building activity. Since the controversy in early Islamic history between the bedouins and the ruling establishment, theologians have emphasized that the Prophet's origin was urban, not bedouin.[367] Al-Jāḥiẓ reports a dialogue that demonstrates, as Ibn Khaldūn centuries later also stressed, that arts and sciences could flourish only in cities; a person who described a village as an agglomeration having a weaver and a teacher received the response, "but that would be a town!"[368]

Authors from the religious establishment also note that shrines and tombs of the saints are all located in cities. Imām Shāfiʿī is said to have warned against rural life as hostile to knowledge and dignity. The Egyptian 16th century mystic Shaʿrānī warned the sufi against country life.[369] The peasants and rural ulema were considered ignorant of Islam because of the absence of proper religious institutions in the provinces. On these grounds, although the *Sharīʿa* prohibits the servitude of Muslims, the Mamluks took the liberty more than once of making slaves of Egyptian peasants and bedouins, arguing that they were not living like proper Muslims.[370] Urbanity is thus rooted in the religion of Islam, which views the human being as a member of a community rather than as a solitary worshiper. Whereas in Europe Bernard de Clairvaux and Petrarch considered the city a corrupt Babylon, for Muslim intellectuals it was the domicile of faith and knowledge.

The *Arabian Nights* includes stories about wealthy cosmopolitan merchants who dealt with goods from all over the world to satisfy a sophisticated clientele. The miniatures of Ḥarīrī's *Maqāmāt*, the most illustrated Arabic book, display urban life in a panoramic perspective showing gatherings in the mosque, the *qadi*'s house, the primary school, the house, the orchard, the bakery, the pharmacy, the barber's shop, and the tavern with musicians. Travels are part of this urban life, they are represented by figures in a tent, or on horse or camel back, or travelling in a boat. The architectural frame is never omitted. Arches are on almost every picture; cupolas and lanterns protrude from the roofs. Architectural decoration, such as elaborate crenellations, *muqarnas*, inscriptions, and arabesques, are always indicated. Despite their sketchy character, the miniatures show houses with furniture: cupboards, shelves, benches and beds, tables with vessels, ornamented cushions and curtains; candlesticks, vases, fruit plates, and jars. It is the same setting that characterizes the bourgeois stories of the *Arabian Nights* from Egypt, Syria, and Iraq. The hero of the *Maqāmāt* is always involved in a gathering where there is a lively conversation. Scenes of eating and drinking are common. A most interesting feature is the fact that each session takes place in a different Muslim city, and since there are altogether fifty sessions, the hero's adventures cover the entire Muslim world.

Building or Architecture?

According to G. Marçais, Islamic architecture developed without the interference of the religious establishment, and therefore the character of architectural conception was secular and profane. The ulema, who included the religious establishment, bureaucrats, and historians and encyclopaedists, received the same kind of education. As has been demonstrated, they were not involved in any conceptualization of the visual arts, although some were poets and literary critics. The medieval historian viewed architecture not in terms of its formal or aesthetic quality, but in terms of its function: monuments were the achievements of monarchs, not of craftsmen, and architecture was history, not art. But the history of art does not necessarily conform to the prevailing ideas on art in a given culture.

The chroniclers of Mamluk Egypt who recorded almost every single day of Egypt's history at that time—an unprecedented and unparalleled undertaking—did not record the name of a single craftsman involved in the building of Sultan Ḥasan's mosque, although they did remark on the outstanding character of the building. The silence of Arabic literature on the identity of craftsmen is all the more remarkable when one considers that a major aspect of Arabic historical literature was the *Ṭabaqāt* or biographical encyclopaedia. The *Ṭabaqāt* literature originated in the early days of Islam as a response to the need to document the life of the Prophet and his companions in a way that would provide guidelines for behavior to the new Muslim community. In time they were expanded to include any notable of Muslim society in the religious ruling and secular establishment. Biographical encyclopaedias document the lives and works of physicians, philosophers, poets, musicians, slave girls, and calligraphers. There are even references to biographies of painters in the 10th century.[371] Building craftsmen, however, do not figure among these groups. Signatures of craftsmen appear more or less frequently at different times and places, but they are more common on portable objects than on buildings.

Plato valued architecture as a creative mathematical discipline that serves order and symmetry and overcomes chaos, and Aristotle saw it as the expression of ideal beauty. Neither considered it among the mimetic arts; therefore it was not discussed in Aristotle's *Poetics*.[372] Medieval European thinkers considered architecture superior to other crafts or *artes mechanicae* because it was based on science.[373] The Arabs, however, did not give it a prominent place in their classification of sciences, nor did they perceive it as a form of art like poetry but rather as a purely functional craft. Historians do speak of building activities, however. The building initiatives of rulers were recorded in chronicles and biographies and mentioned in their obituaries as important features in their careers. It is a characteristic feature of Islamic architecture from India to Morocco to inscribe on the entrance of a building the foundation date and founder's name, thus immortalizing his deed.

Medieval historians dealt with buildings as an administrative or political rather than a creative act, speaking of it in terms of the founder's achievement, or patronage, rather than of the craftsman's. It should be recalled that most of the Muslim architectural heritage consists of religious monuments founded by rulers or by members of the ruling establishment and their closest clientele.

One might be inclined to believe that the Muslim world, like medieval Europe, following the classical tradition, drew a distinction between the mechanical and the liberal arts, but no explicit statements confirm such a discrimination. On the contrary, the term *ṣināʿa* meant technique as well as science and was applied to mechanical as well as intellectual activities. Furthermore, numerous texts stress the importance of acquiring the necessary skills and of mastering the tools of intellectual activities as the artisans do their crafts. An explanation for the absence of reference to craftsmen in Arabic historiography, especially of those involved in the art of building, should be sought in the context of the specific values associated with building. Although other pre-modern cultures did not immortalize their architects either, different patterns and attitudes may be behind the same phenomenon.

Muslim chroniclers described their monarchs as fond of building or deeply involved in the architectural design of their cities and monuments.[374] The caliph al-Manṣūr (754–775) was said to have devised the plan for the round city of Baghdad, and Ibn Ṭūlūn (868–884) was credited with having designed his spiral minaret. The chronicler of Ibn Ṭūlūn does refer to an architect, mentioning that he was a Christian, that he had to spend some time in jail, and that he was generously rewarded for his work, without naming him, however.

The fact that the historian emphasized the role of the ruler and his courtiers as the primary designers of imperial buildings should not be interpreted, however, as mere glorification of the ruler by court historiographers. The majority of medieval Arab historians were not court historians and did not depend directly on rulers; they always had an important margin of freedom. The fact that the historians attributed the creation of a monument to the ruler should rather be related to their view that the erection of a monument was essentially an administrative undertaking. According to Assunto, in medieval Europe the art patron was also the one to whom the credit for the beauty of the art object as well as the responsibility for its deficiencies should be given.[375]

In Muslim society the role of the patron is rooted in the sociopolitical system. Natural resources such as land, water, and minerals were not private property, but theoretically belonged to the entire community. In practice this meant that responsibility for them fell to the ruler and they were subject to his authority. Historians therefore attributed to the ruler the primary responsibility for providing the community with all it needed to fulfill its religious duties, and the ruler was judged accordingly. City planning and building were part of the ruler's duty to ensure the security, welfare, and prosperity of the Muslim community and provide it with adequate means for practicing Islam. Infrastructural works for the pilgrimage and religious and educational institutions belonged to this task, as did all kinds of commercial and civil structures that would contribute to better living standards for the community. It may be important to recall here that the subject of the mosaics adorning the walls of the Umayyad mosque of Damascus is architectural representation. Whatever the symbolism behind these images, buildings have been chosen here to represent something evidently significant enough to be publicized on the walls of the first imperial mosque of Islam. Architecture is associated here with an elevated meaning. The caliph al-Muʿtaṣim is reported to have said that land development or building (*ʿimāra*) had many advantages; it activates land, thus adding life to the world, increases taxes and income, reduces living costs, and allows profit and enterprise to expand.[376]

In a passage in the *Siyāsatnāmeh*, the famous Seljuk mirror of princes, Niẓām al-Mulk wrote of the ruler's duty:

> He should accomplish all works related to the improvement of the world, such as the construction of (hydraulic) *qanāt*s, the digging of major irrigation channels, the building of bridges over great rivers, the development of villages and farms, the erection of fortresses, and the founding of new cities, great monuments, and lofty palaces. He should furthermore build hospices and bases along the caravan roads. Such deeds will perpetuate his name, he will be rewarded in Heaven and prayers will forever be spoken for his sake.[377]

Others have similarly assigned to the monarch the responsibility of building and maintaining cities. Ibn Khaldūn attributes the duty of founding and supervising the Friday mosques and their staff to the ruler.[378] Another 14th-century author equated building with life and ruins with death.[379] At the ruler's death his obituary, the balance sheet of his deeds, would include a list of the buildings he had sponsored.

A dialogue between the 10th-century historian Muqaddasī and his uncle confirms that the foundation of a monument was considered a political act with significant symbolic implications. Muqaddasī told his uncle in his opinion the caliph al-Walīd I (r. 705–715) should have spent money on civic projects such as roads, caravanserais, and fortresses rather than on mosques. The latter answered that the presence of magnificent churches in Syria made it mandatory for Muslim rulers to build splendid mosques, so that the minds of Muslims should not be left to be dazzled only by the splendor of Christian churches.[380] Centuries later, Sultan al-Ẓāhir Baybars, showing his astonishment at the exorbitant sums which one of his amirs spent to build a palace for himself, received the answer, "By God my lord I built this palace so that our enemies may hear about it and say, 'One of the amirs of the Sultan has built such a lavish and expensive house!'"[381] Whether or not this was the real motive is another matter, but the argument, and most of all the fact that it persuaded the sultan, reveals the political meaning associated with the erection of formidable buildings.

According to Ibn Khaldūn building was the oldest and most basic craft;

the quality of the architecture and the degree of its elaboration depended on the power of the rulers and the sophistication of the society.[382] He recognized the importance of princely patronage for religious and intellectual activity, attributing to the state the responsibility not only for economic growth and urban expansion, but also for cultural and intellectual production. The state plays a decisive role in creating a market that attracts the products of sciences and arts. With his statement "People follow the religion of their ruler," Ibn Khaldūn meant that the rulers set the trends of culture and taste.[383] It is interesting to note that in Ibn Shāhīn's (d. ca. 1468) book on the interpretation of dreams, the minaret symbolizes the ruler and royalty and the pulpit both religion and royalty.[384]

Because founding an urban project or a religious building was a moral achievement, the historian attributed the merit of its realization to the founder rather than to the craftsman. Unlike in Europe, the names of architectural styles in the Islamic world are derived from ruling dynasties; this is not an error of Western scholars, but a reflection of the close connection between rulers and the buildings they founded. Unlike medieval cathedrals, most Islamic religious monuments were individual foundations, completed in a very short time during the lifetime of their sponsors, so that the patron could put his personal imprint on his building.

The introductory text of some *waqf* documents includes a statement attributed to the Prophet: "Human beings can perpetuate their deeds beyond death in three ways—by establishing a lasting charity, by conveying useful knowledge, or by giving birth to children who would pray for them." The pious foundation is a lasting charity; it perpetuates the founder's work beyond death. Here it is important to emphasize that the *waqf* (trust) was theoretically unlimited in time. The foundation was supposed to outlive the building and to restore it or rebuild it if necessary. It immortalized the founder by advertising his piety.

In historical accounts a distinction is often made between the religious and functional buildings that served the community, on the one hand, and those built for purely private purposes, on the other. The historian was more interested in the first category. Buildings erected for private use were less relevant to their interests and we are less informed about them. The architectural legacy confirms this distinction between monuments of social relevance and those serving exclusively private interests; in periods of rebellion and war between Muslims, palaces were destroyed but religious buildings were usually spared.

In the biography of Zubayda, Hārūn al-Rashīd's wife, the historian Masʿūdī makes a clear distinction between the serious achievements accomplished by the queen, which included water supply on the pilgrimage road and in the Holy Cities as well as other charitable works, and deeds of a more mundane character, such as innovations in ceremonies and fashions. The monarch, although he was not expected to lead a Spartan life, was supposed to be like a shepherd to his community, not distracted by worldly pleasures.

Monarchs, especially great conquerors and builders, are often reported to have recruited craftsmen from all parts of their empire to build their cities and monuments. Materials and labor that came from remote places enhanced the prestige of the building and of its sponsor. The caliph al-Manṣūr who founded Baghdad, the caliph al-Muʿtaṣim who founded Samarra, Timur in Samarqand, and the Ottoman sultan Selim I are all reported to have taken craftsmen from various places to work in their capitals. As a result, the exploitation of craftsmen by *corvée* and the illegal acquisition of funds for a pious foundation have often been matters of concern to jurists and historians. Maqrīzī describes as "gloomy" the mosques built on confiscated land or by exploited workers. Mamluk scholars even debated the validity of prayer in mosques built with such illicit means. Under the Almoravids in North Africa the dignitaries of Fez chose to enlarge their Great Mosque at their own expense, rather than accept a donation from the ruler, to guarantee that the money was clean.[385] We repeatedly find reports and anecdotes in Muslim chronicles from various periods telling how the founder had taken care to buy the land or made efforts to compensate the owners of land he took for the foundation of his mosque. The allegation, actually a topos, that an ancient treasure had been discovered which enabled the founder to finance his project, was sometimes used to deflect suspicion regarding the source of the funding. Another topos that turns up in chronicles of various periods and places is the refusal of the founder to keep track of expenses for a religious building; because a pious deed should not be subject to calculation, the founder would throw away the receipts presented to him.[386]

Historians are often eloquent when they talk about the first mosques of Islam. Their accounts are full of details and precise information on their original configuration and subsequent enlargements and embellishments. Travelers and pilgrims are also more meticulous than usual when describing the holy mosques of Mecca and Medina or Jerusalem. The earlier their history and the closer to the Prophet and his companions, the more significant the details become. Here, the historian deals not with architectural history, but with history itself.

According to a *ḥadīth* of the Prophet, the shrine at Mecca was older than the temple of Jerusalem founded by Solomon, because it goes back to Abraham, but Ibn Khaldūn says that this refers not to the age of the buildings, but to the tradition of the site as a place of worship.[387] This statement is of great significance because it characterizes the traditional Islamic view of religious monuments as content rather than form. The Kaʿba is perhaps the only monument in Islamic culture that was always restored to look as it originally did. This subject was already being discussed during the Prophet's lifetime, when in the course of a restoration he ordered it to be returned to its original ancient form.

When it came to the holy places, beauty was no longer perceived in terms of aesthetic pleasure, but in terms of religious pleasure. A 15th-century author writes that God looks at Jerusalem with the eye of beauty, whereas he looks at Mecca with the eye of majesty. Therefore Jerusalem is agreeable, wide, and beautiful (*bahja, saʿa, manẓar ḥasan*), but the shrine at Mecca is august, elegant, and formidable (*ubbaha, waqār, hayba*).[388] The 12th-century traveler Ibn Jubayr describes a *madrasa* as a *maʾnasa* (place of enjoyment), and Maqrīzī describes mosques in similar terms as places of recreation and enjoyment (*muntazah, uns*), thus associating learning and worship with pleasure. In a reference to Cairo's cemetery, Maqrīzī uses similar words, *ṭarab* and *muntazah*, mentioning moonlight and gatherings in the context of shrines and sanctuaries. At night when the moon shines and music fills the air the cemetery attracts both the devout and the hedonist.[389]

Muslim historians looked upon pre-Islamic monuments as documents and lessons in history and endowed them with moral value. The monuments were admired as products of past cultures that possessed enormous wisdom and knowledge. Masʿūdī ascribed to ancient kings the merit of introducing and sponsoring the sciences and arts, combining knowledge with power.[390] In ancient societies religion and royal power were interdependent.

In his introduction to the description of the pyramids of Egypt, the 13th-century historian Idrīsī cites various texts from the Koran admonishing people to look around the world, so that they can learn wisdom and morality from past events. Idrīsī adds that "wondering about wonderful things is a sign of the intellect's health and vitality."[391] "Whoever builds a structure that is destined to remain; when his name is inscribed therein, for as long as the structure lasts, that name will be on the lips of people."[392]

About the same time an Egyptian poet said:

Memory of kings' ambitions after they're gone
in their buildings is nourished;
look at the pyramids still standing
after their kings have perished;
if the monument is great
it tells of great goals now vanished.[393]

And Ibn Iyās, referring to the building activities of the amir Azbak in the 15th century, wrote, "A knight does not enjoy the shine of chivalry unless he bequeaths a monument on earth."[394]

Another poet deplored the suffering of monuments damaged by vandalism and exclaimed:

Vandal, may your right hand be crippled!
leave them for the one who sees, asks and beholds,
houses of people tell stories,
No better stories than tales of abodes.[395]

The historian Ibn Marzūq condemned those responsible for the neglect and destruction of historical monuments, and promised that God would judge and punish them, "because they deleted symbols that are a source of pride and honor to the Muslims over time."[396]

Ibn Khaldūn revered and admired the monuments of pre-Islamic cultures, seeing in their magnificence a testimony to the greatness of these cultures that produced them.[397] They were the merit of the entire society that contributed to their creation over generations. Comparing the ancient monuments with the buildings of his own time, he criticized the individualistic character of Muslim rulers who each preferred to erect his own monument rather than maintain or complete a project began by his predecessors.

Admiration for the ancient monuments simultaneously acknowledged their superiority to contemporary buildings. The pyramids, for example, were praised as the greatest architectural achievements on earth. One of the most interesting descriptions of ancient Egyptian monuments in Arabic literature is the account of ʿAbd al-Laṭīf al-Baghdādī, a physician and scholar of the 12th century whose comments on the art of earlier monuments with references to their shape, their proportions, their orientation and geometry, the freshness of their colors, and the quality of their craftsmanship are enthusiastic, even passionate. He admired the artist who sculpted the sphinx of Giza for having been able to observe proportionality on such a colossal scale: the statue "seems to smile gently"; the marvels of the temples of Memphis confound the mind: the more one looks at them, the more one's fascination increases.[398] ʿAbd al-Laṭīf writes that the Egyptian monuments were conceived not just for pleasure, but in order to convey an important message to posterity. He goes on to say that past Muslim generations had been careful to preserve these monuments because they were equivalent to chronicles of past cultures; since these cultures are mentioned in the Koran they thus confirm the words of God. With this argument, ʿAbd al-Laṭīf strongly condemned those who damaged the monuments while searching for gold. We find such condemnation in other sources as well: Ibn Khaldūn and Ibn Iyās note bitterly that it is easier to demolish than to build. Another scholar wrote of the pyramids:

> They tell about the strength of their people and report their deeds, they speak of their knowledge and their minds, and narrate their deeds and history.[399]

The use of verbs like "speak," "tell," and "narrate" (*tuḥaddith, tanṭaq,* and *tukhbir*) emphasizes the documentary function of architecture. The Pharos of Alexandria has been frequently described (partly relying on old accounts) with an almost exceptional care for detail. Nostalgia for the architecture of the past as superior to the present is always implied in a didactic and moralizing tone, even when the past is not so remote. One of the Mamluk sultans of the 15th century tried unsuccessfully to destroy the mosque of Sultan Ḥasan because rebels had entrenched themselves in it in order to shoot at the residence of the sultan in the Citadel. Ibn Iyās ridiculed the operation, using the occasion to praise the high quality of the old craftsmanship, which the workers of his time were not even able to destroy.

The value of a monument as a historical record was acknowledged equally by historians and rulers. Jāḥiẓ wrote that the Persians' greatest achievement was architecture and that the Arabs were equally proficient in this field, but their greatest talent lay in literature. The first lines of the book on *Beauties and Antitheses*, attributed to him, are dedicated to a comparison between the cultural values of architecture and literature. Although he concludes with a preference for literature because of its durability, Jāḥiẓ acknowledged the documentary value of architecture as medium for the rulers to propagate their achievements, as the Persians did with their rock carvings.[400] Other authors believed that the ancient monuments had been erected as repositories for the science and knowledge of the ancient Egyptians, which were carved on the walls to save them from decay.

In one of the academic gatherings held by the Mamluk sultan al-Ghūrī, one of the scholars mentioned Sultan Maḥmūd of Ghazna (11th century), who when seeking ways to immortalize his name was advised to erect monuments; he responded that the monuments would not last more than a few centuries and decided instead to sponsor the *Shāhnāmeh* of Firdawsī.[401]

The weighing of the monument against the book is a topos. The medieval Muslim was well aware of the fact that the quest for immortality was a major motive for rulers to establish pious foundations. Even if preference was ultimately given to the book, the monument was a document in stone that was more visible and thus of more immediate effect. If the book was documentation, the monument was advertisement. Maḥmūd of Ghazna and Sultan al-Ghūrī used both to perpetuate their name; Maḥmūd sponsored the compilation of the *Shāhnāmeh* and al-Ghūrī sponsored its first translation into Turkish. In a society where statues or portraits of the monarchs were not allowed, this kind of patronage was of particular significance. One of the reasons why Muslims equated architecture with history is the very fact that Islam took root in regions with an extremely rich historical and cultural heritage, often manifested in the form of monuments rather than through legible sources. Monarchs' eagerness to have their names associated with monuments sometimes led to cases of imposture. The Abbasid caliph al-Maʾmūn inscribed his name on the Dome of the Rock instead of that of the founder ʿAbd al-Malik (685–705)—although he did not, and could not, fake the history of the monument, he wanted his name inscribed on it. The caliph al-Mahdī (775–785) is said to have been so eager to have his name on buildings along the pilgrimage road that he even tried to inscribe it on buildings erected by others, in exchange for financial compensation.[402] Al-Nāṣir Muḥammad eradicated the name of Amir Baybars al-Jashankīr from the *khanqāh* he had built, to punish him for having tried to usurp the throne. This does not mean that he denied that Baybars ever built the *khanqāh*; he could have destroyed more fragile evidence, in the form of the foundation deed, but he did not, and historians continued to attribute the foundation to Baybars. The punishment consisted in removing his name from the building. Sultan al-Nāṣir was even accused by some chroniclers of having demolished buildings erected by his predecessors and rebuilt them just to have his own name commemorated instead of theirs.

One of the most effective methods for a monarch to perpetuate his name was to attach his mausoleum to his religious foundation. Whereas the foundation of the first cathedral mosques was part of the conquest and Islamization of the territory to which the entire community contributed, the mosques of the later period were not anonymous. With the spread of the *madrasa*, the *khanqāh*, and the neighborhood mosque, to which the mausoleum of the founder was often attached, the religious foundation became increasingly associated with the name of its founder. The political character of architecture is confirmed by the prominent place occupied by historical epigraphy, which indicates the sponsor's name and the foundation date. Such inscriptions are usually found on facades, most often on the portal, as an announcement to visitors.

The architecture of past cultures, like their traditions, was integrated into Islamic heritage because of the nature of Islam and the Koran, which acknowledged and adopted biblical traditions. Even Greek mythological figures were identified with biblical prophets. The Kaʿba is believed to have been built by Abraham and the Dome of the Rock, the first great monument of Islam, was erected on a holy biblical site. Muḥammad was *khātim al-anbiyāʾ*, the last and concluding prophet. He confirmed and crowned the message of his predecessors to make Islam the perfect end to the sequence of monotheistic religions. Since Islamic culture flourished in territories where these religious traditions had originated, cultural continuity was a principle of Islamic politics. All important Muslim cemeteries in Egypt, Syria, and Mesopotamia were associated with legends relating the site to biblical and Christian traditions.

Monuments were often regarded as part of the booty captured in war, like the craftsmen deported from conquered territories. An often related story is that Hārūn al-Rashīd was dissuaded from destroying the Sasanian palace of Ctesiphon, admired by the Arabs as a wonder of architecture, by his counselors' suggestion that he leave the monument as a memorial and evidence of the superiority of the Arabs who had succeeded in defeating a nation great enough to erect such grand building!

The Arabic poets of the Crusades period, to celebrate the booty that fell into Muslim hands, emphasized the great beauty of the Christian women and the magnificence of the buildings constructed by their enemies the Crusaders. By praising the enemy's achievements, they celebrated their own triumph. Maqrīzī, for example, regarded the portal of the *madrasa* of al-Nāṣir Muḥammad to be one of the greatest in the world;[403] Cairo at that time had other portals much more impressive in size and craftsmanship, but this one was a trophy taken from a Crusaders' church in Palestine; it was therefore a symbol of Muslim triumph and consequently beautiful. Sultan Baybars built a monumental dome over the prayer niche of his mosque, the largest of its kind in Cairo, with materials captured in his campaigns against the Crusaders. The beauty and quality of the trophy is a tribute to the winner; it is a symbol of his power.

In descriptions of cities, function and performance were the essential criteria; Islamic culture had no formal rules for planning a city. In the geographical literature of the classical age, a city was judged in terms of its impregnability, its clean air, its water supply, the fertility of its agricultural hinterland; other important criteria included the size and importance of the markets, the prices and supply of goods, and the number of baths. In the later period scholars and their institutions were also regarded as assets to a city. When the 15th-century historian al-ʿAynī praised Maqrīzī's description of Cairo, he wrote, "He gave life to her monuments, shed light on her mysteries, revived her legacy, and portrayed her notables."[404] The activities of the city, rather than its formal features, were what mattered.

A 9th-century poem cited by Masʿūdī, mourning the destruction of Baghdad after a civil war, also reflects the same idea, that a city was judged by the quality of life it provided.

> O Baghdad city of kings, goal of all desires,
> Center of all learnings of Islam,
> Paradise on earth, you who sought wealth and gave
> Birth to hope in every merchant's breast,
> Tell us, where are they whom we once met
> Along pleasure's flowery roads?
> Where are the kings, shining amidst their trains
> Like brilliant stars?
> Where are the qadis, resolving by reason's light
> The conundrums of the Law?
> Where are the preachers and poets with their wisdom,
> Speaking harmonious words?
> Where are your gardens rich in charm, the palaces
> Along the river banks, the flourishing land?
> Where are the royal pavilions I once knew,
> Glittering with jewels? Once
> The earth was sprinkled with musk and rose,
> The smoke of incense spread far and wide.
> Every night the joyful guests gathered
> At the home of some noble and generous host.
> He gave orders and the singing girls
> Raised their beautiful voices and married
> Them to the sound of the flute in a song.
> Where have they gone, those glorious kings?[405]

No reference is made to the plan of the city or style of its architecture; only the quality of life is praised and its disappearance deplored. The values of Baghdad lay with its merchants, *qadi*s, poets, preachers, musicians. When the poem does refer to palaces, gardens, and pavilions, it is only as metaphors for a glamorous style of life.

Al-Jāḥiẓ's descriptions of Basra and Kufa mention climate, terrain, the hunt, water, the fruits, and the markets. In an anecdote from the *Kitāb al-Aghānī*, when the poet Ḥammād praised the city of Ḥīra to his friends he spoke of its fresh air, sweet water, and beautiful landscape, but his friends remained skeptical. To persuade them, Ḥammād invited them to a banquet, offering meats, wines, and fruits from Ḥīra served in vessels and on furniture made in that city. The servants also came from Ḥīra, as did the poetry the host recited to his guests. In the end the guests were willing to acknowledge the virtues of Ḥīra.[406]

In a 16th-century poem composed to lament the desertion of a Nile island that had once been popular as a summer resort and place of entertainment, the poet bemoaned the loss of trees and birds, the mosque and palaces, vendors of sweetmeats, cheese, fruits, and flowers. Even the hashish-eater and the wine drinker were missed, along with singers and musicians, as part of the carefree life that had vanished.[407]

Just as the city is judged according to the quality of life it offers, so buildings were often valued in terms of their functions. Though the historians say little about stylistic or technical innovations such as the first appearance of a certain plan, whenever innovations are mentioned, it is for their political and religious significance rather than for their stylistic quality. Historians might praise a structure's size, or the value of the material used and the quality of the workmanship, but statements on the originality of a design were always vague. Although Maqrīzī was the author of the most comprehensive medieval source on the topography and monuments of Cairo, he was badly informed about architecture and architects; he described a minaret as the first in Cairo to be built in stone, when there were extant examples to show that it had several predecessors![408]

If we had available written statements by a sponsor comparable to those made by Abbot Suger of St. Denis in France, we would have a different image of the monuments. The aesthetic concepts of the designers of architecture are absent from the picture presented by the historian. But the sponsors and the craftsmen of the Arab world did not write about themselves; they were not intellectuals. Those who articulated ideas and concepts were the ulema who, though they often depended on official sponsorship, were not enslaved by it, as the rulers needed the ulema's

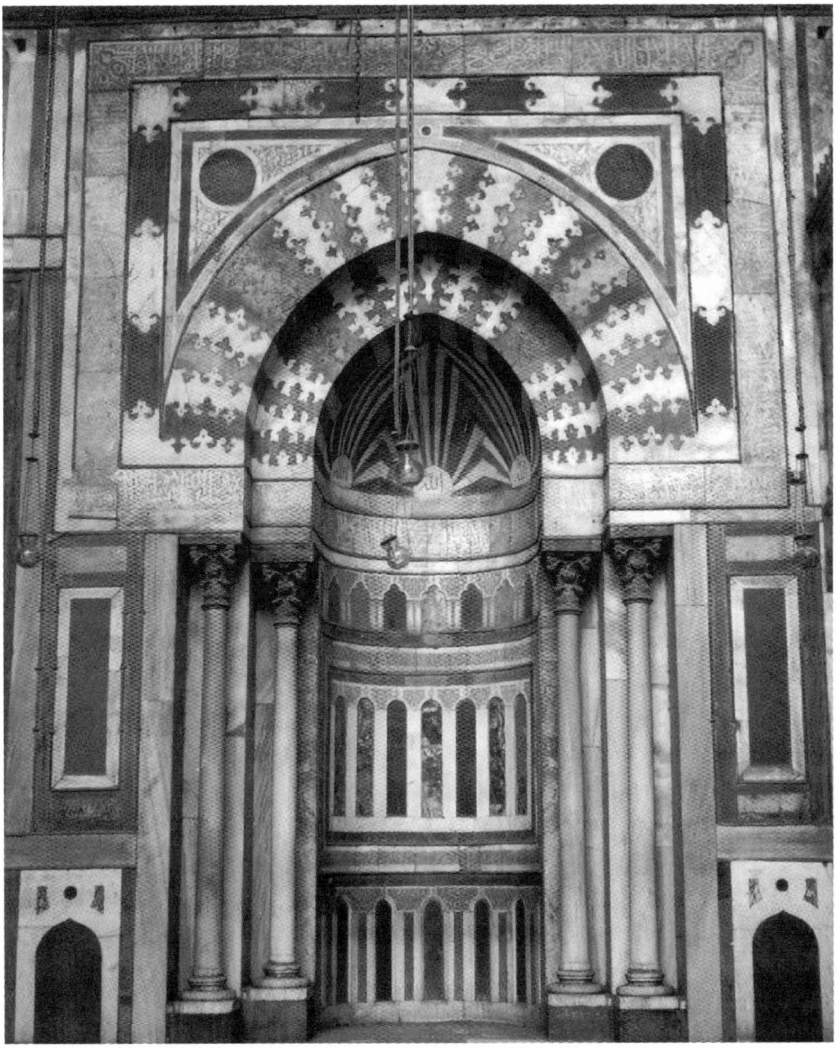

Prayer niche (*miḥrāb*) at the mosque of Sultan Ḥasan, Cairo, 14th c.

support for their own legitimation.

Unlike the Gothic cathedral, whose architecture owed as much to the religious philosophy of an epoch as to its craftsmen and sponsors, Islamic religious architecture was designed entirely by laymen, viz. patrons, administrators, and craftsmen; theorists left the aesthetics of architecture to its patrons and practitioners. The strong grip of the ruling establishment on the building craft and the identification of the ruler's image with architecture, on the one hand, and the absence of building craftsmen in the circle of the ulema on the other, must have had important consequences on the status of this craft. It could also have been what prevented the economic emancipation of the building craft and the conceptualization of architecture as an art in its own right.

The picture conveyed by medieval historians did not tell the whole story of architecture, but it did reveal an important aspect of its meaning to contemporary society. Because of its close connection to the ruling establishment and its patronage, architecture was of political and historical concern. It is not surprising that ʿAbd al-Laṭīf's description of Egypt is called *al-ifāda wa'l-iʿtibār* (edification and lesson), Maqrīzī's descriptions of Egypt's cities and their monuments *al-mawāʿiẓ wa'l-iʿtibār fī'l-khiṭaṭ wa 'l-āthār* (the morality and lesson in the history of places and monuments), and Ibn Khaldūn's world history *kitāb al-ʿibar* (the book of lessons).

Conclusion

The modern concept of aesthetics, based on the ideas of 18th-century philosophers such as Baumgarten, Hume, and Kant, focuses on the aesthetic experience and views aesthetic beauty as autonomous, to be valued for itself. It is uncommitted to moral or religious values and does not identify the beautiful with the good. Although Aristotle distinguished between beauty for pleasure and moral beauty, classical and medieval Western concepts of beauty generally gravitated toward the Platonic approach of linking the beautiful with the good. Because of its association with moral values, Christian theologians included beauty as a topic in their theological discourse. As we have seen, the mainstream of Arabic Islamic thought tended rather to the peripatetic approach, which allowed the development of autonomous norms of beauty that were independent of moral or religious criteria. The artistic work was viewed separately from the divine scheme and was free of metaphysical associations.

Beauty, however, had a significant place in religious thought. The Arab-Muslim tradition views the beauty of the universe, emphasized in the Koran, and the literary superiority of the Koranic text itself as a compelling evidence for the divine hand. Under the influence of Greek thought, philosophers, sufis, and theologians dealt with the beauty-love relationship as the basic factor in the motion of the universe. Sufi worship is based on passion for God's beauty which is manifest in the human image, created to resemble God's.

The principle that Islam is not only binding on the individual but also on the whole society (*dunyā wa dīn*), encompassing worship (*ʿibādāt*) as well as social behavior (*muʿāmalāt*), did not prevent the formation of a profane culture. Islamic law did acknowledge the existence of a domain it cannot rule directly, but only indirectly, through the principles of common interest (*maṣlaḥa*). This resulted in the articulation of the ruler's domain or *siyāsa*. The rational sciences, which belonged to the Greek heritage, continued to be part of the Islamic academic repertoire even after philosophy was discarded by orthodoxy, and they were taught in mosques and *madrasas* throughout the entire pre-modern epoch. Profane culture, to which the arts belonged, had its acknowledged place as long as it did not conflict with the *Sharīʿa*.

Having created a huge empire on the territory of the great ancient civilizations, the Arab conquerors saw themselves as the heirs of these cultures and acted accordingly as great patrons of the arts. Greek and Persian models were referred to in court ceremonial. The sponsorship of the arts, which bestowed a brilliance on the monarchs, was viewed as beneficial to the image of the Muslim community when facing its Christian antagonists.

Muslim doctrine assigns to the ruler the task of providing the community with an adequate religious, social, and urban environment. Princely patronage guided all religious and cultural activities. The monarchs and their entourage were also the ones who sponsored the religious institutions in the big cities and appointed their superiors. The absence of a clerical institution in Sunni Muslim society prevented the articulation of a sacral art dictated by religious criteria, as it existed in medieval Europe. It was the ruling, not the religious, establishment who decided what mosques should look like.

Poetry, calligraphy, music, architecture, and the decorative arts flourished under the sponsorship of the ruling establishment. Urban growth and the prosperity of the urban bourgeoisie were a major achievement under Islam, but the cities were not autonomous or rivals to the royal court. The city was the center of power, of religion, and of art. Arab-Islamic culture was urban and Arabic literature did not acknowledge the vernacular.

Because poetry was the supreme, most widespread, and most discussed art of the medieval Arab world, concepts of beauty are mainly to be found there. They were articulated by poets, literary critics, and philosophers. Although literary criticism was an offshoot of the religious science, of Koranic exegesis, poetry was not in the domain of religion. It was Muslim orthodoxy itself, based on the Prophet's distance from the poets, that let this art go its profane way. Religious poetry was honored less than profane poetry.

Arabic literary criticism observed the Aristotelian distinction between content and form; the quality of an artistic work and its potential for producing pleasure depend primarily on the artist's intelligence and skill in execution, rather than on the work's content, meaning, or originality. No metaphysical powers are involved in artistic creation. This principle confirmed the non-sacral orientation of the arts; Sufi poets adopted the vocabulary of erotic and bacchic poetry to address God, and craftsmen applied the same architectural and decorative idiom to religious and to profane monuments.

Ibn Sīnā recognized the uncommitted, pleasure-oriented character of Arabic poetry, and most critics regarded good poetry as that without any didactic purpose. The prevailing attitude in literary criticism and philosophy was that poetry should be impressive and pleasing, not narrative or informative as in the Greek and Iranian tradition. Narrative arts were identified as purposeful and didactic, whereas abstractness was associated with pleasure.

In music virtuosity was associated with diabolic rather than divine inspiration. Music, poetry, and wine belonged to the same category of hedonistic experience. Musicology was inherited from the Greeks and integrated in the repertoire of Muslim sciences, but music in its social context was a source of controversy because of its licentious associations. In response to the puritans, Ghazālī argued that poetry and music cannot *per se* be bad, but only their licentious use. This is an acknowledgement that the arts were autonomous; their moral value was a matter of subjective application. Wine poetry continued to be composed in the Arab world until the late Ottoman period, and music was acknowledged by the sufis to be a source of ecstasy which brings man closer to God.

Among the visual arts, only calligraphy had the status of an academic discipline. What modern art historians identify as characteristic Islamic design was not formulated as such by its creators. There was no explicit discussion among Arab medieval authors of what distinguished the Islamic visual arts from the arts of other cultures, aside from hostility to figural representations. The aesthetics of geometry and abstract vegetal motifs in Islamic design were not articulated or verbalized in any kind of literature. The usefulness of mathematics and its didactic effect were emphasized, but without discussing the aesthetic aspects of geometry so prominently displayed in Islamic art.

The Prophet is reported to have said in a *ḥadīth* that "everything has its ornament." But according to another *ḥadīth*, the Prophet was hostile to lavish architecture. As in many other instances presented in this study, different, contradictory trends co-existed. The ulema did not discuss any visual art. Their hostility toward figural representation was not a matter of canonical prohibition; the firmest statements on this subject were made in a late period, after Islamic art had already acquired its basic features.

There is no evidence in Arabic sources to suggest any religious symbolic meaning attributed to Islamic design, whether to the arabesque or geometry. Grabar's emphasis on the pleasure-oriented nature of Islamic design can be confirmed. The creation of the visual arts was guided by aesthetic criteria alone; as an expression of beauty, the art object could serve as a religious or a status symbol, or to embellish everyday life.

Inscriptions adorned all kinds of objects, just as poetry celebrated all things including cuisine. Nothing escaped elaboration and stylization. There was no religious prohibition against representing a tree or a flower in a naturalistic manner, but the Arab artist preferred stylization. Naturalistic motifs are much rarer in Arab than in Iranian or Turkish art. In later periods this tendency increased.

Architecture occupies a singular place in literature. It was defined neither as a scientific discipline nor as an art equivalent to painting, which was often compared to poetry and associated with imagination. The historians, our main source on building activities, although they do mention the pleasure of looking at handsome buildings, focus their interest rather on their functional aspect. Monuments were viewed according to their relevance to public interest, and were associated with statecraft, as expressions of the ruler's devotion and sense of duty. The meaning associated with architecture was thus social and political. Its aesthetic criteria were set by the craftsmen and their patrons and are documented only in the works themselves.

If Arabic culture did not elaborate a general theory of aesthetic, Arabic thinkers between the 10th and the 12th centuries did, however, develop concepts dealing with the artistic work and the perception of beauty that focused on knowledge and endeavor as the basis for the creation of art as well as for its enjoyment.

The originality of the Arabic discourse on beauty lies in its emphasis on the psychological factor of delectability. Beauty is measured by the degree of pleasure it incites in the recipient; the individual capacity for appreciation, which follows psychological needs, can be highly sharpened. The individual, however, is addressed as a member of a society where norms are set and knowledge is cultivated.

At the end of the 14th century, Ibn Khaldūn, the last great and original Arab thinker before pre-modern times, added a new dimension to the rationalistic approach to the arts by linking all cultural activities to the political and social environment. However, the modernity anticipated in Ibn Khaldūn's thought provoked no intellectual breakthroughs. Stagnation characterized the culture of the following centuries. The heritage faithfully conserved through the period of political decline continued to be cherished, as time passed, as reminiscence of a golden age.

Notes

1. Kahwaji, "ʿIlm al-Djamāl," *E.I.*[2]
2. "Si les auteurs du moyen âge n'ont guère de théorie systématisée des beaux-arts, ce n'est pas qu'ils ignorent les rapports entre l'art et la beauté." De Bruyne, p. 221.
3. Arberry, *Revelation*, p. 62.
4. Arnaldez, "Maʿrifa," *E.I.*[2]
5. See Rosenthal's *Knowledge Triumphant.*
6. Lewis, "Siyasa"; Busse, "Fürstenspiegel."
7. von Grunebaum, *Kritik*, p. 129.
8. Hillenbrand, p. 264, quoting Wensinck.
9. Rosenthal, *Four Essays*, p. 12
10. Abu Deeb, *Jurjani*, pp. 24ff.
11. "Gott ist schön," *Frankfurter Allgemeine Zeitung*, 8 June 1996.
12. Ibn Qayyim, *Rawḍa*, p. 253.
13. Dols, p. 297.
14. Arkoun, *Traité*, pp. 133ff.
15. *shahīd,* usually translated "martyr," is a person who is killed in a holy war, for the victory of Islam.
16. Koran quotations, unless otherwise noted, are taken from the translation by N.J. Dawood (London: Penguin, 1990).
17. Also 37:6–7, 15:16, and 41:11–12.
18. For Ghazālī's statements on beauty and love, see *Iḥyāʾ,* IV, pp. 99ff., 117f., 270–90, 396ff., 495; Hillenbrand, "Ghazali"; Ettinghausen, "Ghazzali"; Ritter, *Elixier*, pp. 187ff.
19. Ghazālī, III, p. 380.
20. Ghazālī, III, p. 97.
21. Ettinghausen's translation; Ghazālī, IV, p. 275.
22. Ettinghausen, "Ghazzali," p. 164.
23. Ghazālī, III, p. 20f., VI, p. 156.
24. Arberry, *Avicenna*, pp. 64ff.
25. Ghazālī, IV, p. 273.
26. Ibn Qayyim, *Rawḍa*, p. 160.
27. Ibn Qayyim, *Rawḍa*, pp. 65ff.; 176.
28. Arberry, *Saints*, p. 47.
29. See Massignon, *Passion*.
30. Arberry, *Aspects*, p. 218.
31. Arberry, *Aspects*, p. 66.
32. Nicholson, *Literary History*, p. 397
33. Fakhry, p. 261.

34. Fakhry, p. 166.
35. Ikhwān al-Ṣafā, III, p. 280.
36. Nasr, pp. 44f.
37. Ibid.
38. Fakhry, p. 142.
39. Fakhry, pp. 264f.
40. Affifi, p. 173.
41. Corbin, *Ibn ʿArabi*, p. 78.
42. Corbin, *Ibn ʿArabi*, p. 205.
43. Ghazālī, IV, p. 312.
44. Nicholson, *Mystics*, p. 112.
45. Nicholson's translation, *Mystics*, p. 103.
46. Homerin, p. 11.
47. Ibn Qayyim, *Rawḍa*, pp. 99f.
48. Fakhry, p. 159.
49. Not to be confused with Ibn Ṭufayl's later narrative mentioned above, which also uses the name Ḥayy b. Yaqẓān.
50. Arnaldez, "Ibn Rushd," *E.I.*[2]
51. Arberry, *Way*, p. 74.
52. Affifi, pp. 124f.
53. Fakhry, p. 248.
54. Saʿd, pp. 280ff.
55. Both passages in Arberry, *Way*, p. 70.
56. Ikhwān al-Ṣafā, I, pp. 253f.; III, p. 469.
57. Ikhwān al-Ṣafā, I, pp. 80, 103; Nasr, p. 45.
58. Nasr, pp. 45f.
59. Biruni, *Gärten*, pp. 42f.
60. Pellat, *Geisteswelt*, p. 421.
61. De Sacy, pp. 186–96; Maqrīzī, I, p. 122.
62. Ibn Qayyim, *Rawḍa*, p. 229.
63. Jurjānī, pp. 153, 154.
64. Abu Deeb, *Jurjani*, p. 282; Jurjani, p. 150.
65. Ibn Khaldūn, *Muqaddima*, pp. 470f.
66. Sabra, I, pp. 200–207.
67. Sabra, I, p. 201.
68. Tatarkievicz, II, pp. 263–71.
69. Sabra, I, pp. 200ff.
70. Geries, p. 55.
71. Pellat, *Geisteswelt*, p. 222.
72. Pellat, *Geisteswelt*, p. 420.
73. Ghazālī, IV, pp. 296f.
74. Goichon, *Directives*, pp. 470ff.
75. Abu Deeb, *Jurjani*, p. 278; Jurjānī, pp. 133f.
76. Iṣbahānī, VI, p. 117.
77. Nicholson, *Literary History*, p. 309.
78. De Bruyne, p. 32.

79. Eco, p. 119.
80. De Bruyne, pp. 225f.
81. 1) soundness of the human body, 2) soundness of the senses, 3) soundness of the capacity for knowing how to discern what leads to the soundness of the body and the senses, and 4) soundness of the power to labor at what leads to their soundness. Mahdi, *Alfarabi*, p. 71.
82. Mahdi, *Alfarabi*, p. 73; ʿUṣfūr, *Qirāʾa*, pp. 277f.
83. Gardet, "Djanna," *E.I.*[2]
84. ʿAbd al-Raḥmān, pp. 332f.
85. Ettinghausen & Grabar, p. 34.
86. Duri, "Baghdad," *E.I.*[2]
87. Hamori, p. 79.
88. Abu Nuwās, p. 692.
89. *Arabian Nights* (tr. Haddawy), "The Story of Nur al-Din Ali Ibn Bakkar and the Slave Girl Shams al-Nahar," p. 298.
90. *Arabian Nights* (tr. Haddawy), p. 130.
91. *Arabian Nights* (tr. Haddawy), p. 131.
92. Sourdel, *Civilisation*, p. 356.
93. von Grunebaum, *Kritik*, p. 68.
94. Elisseeff, p. 136.
95. Ibn Sīrīn (attr.), pp. 345ff.; Ibn Shāhīn, II, p. 6.
96. Arberry, *Aspects*, p. 22.
97. Lunde & Stone, pp. 403f.
98. Grünert, p. 4.
99. *Arabian Nights* (tr. Haddawy), p. 173.
100. Ibn Qayyim, *Rawḍa*, pp. 239ff.
101. See Ghazālī, III, pp. 97ff.
102. Vadet, p. 43.
103. Nicholson, *Literary History*, p. 106.
104. Ibn Qayyim, *Rawḍa*, p. 228.
105. Ibn Qayyim, *Rawḍa*, pp. 240–44.
106. Sadan, Rainhart, Reinert, "Shaʿr," *E.I.*[2]
107. Arazi, "Al-Shayb wa'l-Shabāb," *E.I.*[2]
108. *Arabian Nights* (tr. Haddawy) pp. 118, 117.
109. *Arabian Nights* (tr. Haddawy) p. 139.
110. *Arabian Nights* (tr. Haddawy) p. 138.
111. *Arabian Nights* (tr. Haddawy) p. 346.
112. Littmann, VI, 2, pp. 379ff. The motif of seduction from a portrait is of Iranian origin.
113. Miquel, p. 198.
114. Ibn Qayyim, *Rawḍa*, p. 229.
115. Iṣbahānī, XVI, p. 160.
116. Iṣbahānī, X, p. 162.
117. Iṣbahānī, X, p. 177.
118. Sellheim, "Lächeln."
119. Müller, *Sklavenkauf*.

120. Iṣbahānī, II, p. 360, V, p. 340.
121. Ibn Qayyim, *Rawḍa*, p. 217.
122. Ghazālī, IV, p. 99.
123. Ibn Qayyim, *Rawḍa*, p. 219.
124. Ibn Qayyim, *Rawḍa*, p. 215.
125. Abū Ḥayyān, *Muqābasāt*, p. 226.
126. Ibn Qayyim, *Rawḍa*, pp. 117, 127f.
127. Van Gelder, p. 63.
128. Arberry, *Aspects*, pp. 187f.; Ibn Ḥazm, p. 109f.
129. Ibn Khaldūn, *Muqaddima,* pp. 470f.
130. C. Brockelmann and J. Vernet, "al-Anṭākī," *E.I.*[2]
131. Masʿūdī, II, pp. 354ff., 518f.; Lunde & Stone, pp. 109f.
132. Pellat, *Geisteswelt*, p. 425.
133. Corbin, *Philosophie*, p. 314.
134. Vadet, p. 388ff.
135. Arberry, *Aspects*, p. 178 (with the author's modification); Ibn Ḥazm, p. 59.
136. Ibn Qayyim, *Rawḍa*, pp. 109, 155.
137. Ibn Qayyim, *Rawḍa*, p. 211.
138. Ibn Qayyim, *Rawḍa*, p. 173f.
139. On this subject see Khairallah.
140. Khairallah, p. 78.
141. Arberry, *Aspects*, p. 122.
142. Arberry, *Aspects*, p. 127.
143. Ibn Qayyim, *Rawḍa*, p. 163.
144. Ibn Qayyim, *Ṭibb*, p. 233.
145. Ibn Qayyim, *Ṭibb*, pp. 233f.
146. Ibn Qayyim, *Ṭibb*, p. 234.
147. On this subject see Farmer, "al-Kindī."
148. Masʿūdī, II, p. 591.
149. Berque, pp. 38, 42f.
150. Ikhwān al-Ṣafā, I, p. 289.
151. Nawājī, p. 178.
152. al-ʿAbbāsī, pp. 14, 122ff.
153. Farmer, "al-Kindī," p. 37.
154. Shiloah, p. 212.
155. Ibn Khaldūn, *Muqaddima*, pp. 469–75.
156. Shiloah, pp. 42f.
157. Ghazālī, II, p. 249; During, "Grincement," p. 166.
158. Vadet, p. 79.
159. During, *Musique*, pp. 42f.
160. Ghazālī, II, p. 245–80; III, p. 120; V, pp. 110–23.
161. Farmer, "The Influence of Music," p. 91.
162. Ibid.
163. ʿUṣfūr, *Qiraʾa*, p. 325.
164. Abū Ḥayyān, *Imtāʿ*, I, p. 214.
165. Abū Ḥayyān, *Muqābasāt*, p. 102.

166. Iṣbahānī, V, pp. 375f.
167. Iṣbahānī, I, p. 4.
168. Shiloah, p. 9.
169. Nawājī, p. 180.
170. Iṣbahānī, V, p. 326.
171. Shiloah, p. 43.
172. Pellat, "ḳayna," *E.I.*[2]
173. Littmann, IV, 2, pp. 645–59.
174. Iṣbahānī, V, p. 230.
175. Sawa, p. 188.
176. al-Faruqi, "Ornamentation," pp. 26f.
177. al-Faruqi, p. 20.
178. Iṣbahānī, V, p. 340.
179. "le principe social par excellence, discipline, politesse et idéal, par lequel l'individu s'affirme comme membre d'un groupe." Vadet, p. 327.
180. Gabrieli, "Adab," *E.I.*[2]
181. Masʿūdī, *Murūj al-dhahab*; trans. Lunde & Stone, *Meadows of Gold. The Abbasids.*
182. Lunde & Stone, *Meadows of Gold*, p. 378; Masʿūdī, *Murūj al-dhahab*, II, p. 647.
183. Heine, pp. 12–26.
184. Heine, p. 25.
185. Arberry, *Aspects*, p. 160; Masʿūdī, II, p. 714. *Miṭrāf* is a kind of shawl.
186. Arberry, *Aspects*, pp. 163f.; Masʿūdī, II, p. 717.
187. Lunde & Stone, p. 377; Masʿūdī, II, p. 645.
188. Arkoun, "Islamic Culture," p. 15.
189. Bosworth I, pp. 31ff.
190. Bencheich, "Khamriyya," *E.I.*[2]
191. Ḥilmī, pp. 37ff.
192. Nicholson, *Literary History,* p.318.
193. Van Gelder, p. 63.
194. Trabulsi, pp. 119ff.
195. Buttersworth, p. 140; Van Gelder, p. 101.
196. ʿAbbās, pp. 38f.; Van Gelder, p. 42.
197. ʿUṣfūr, *Ṣūra*, p. 68.
198. Goodman, p. 226.
199. Dahiyat, pp. 48f., 74.
200. Goodman, p. 223
201. Arberry, *Aspects*, pp. 256f.
202. W. Walter in her afterword to Rückert, *Hariri*, p. 285.
203. Maqrīzī, *Khiṭaṭ*, I, pp. 118f.; Idrīsī/Haarmann, pp. 145f.
204. Iṣbahānī, I, p. 2
205. Rosenthal, *Fortleben*, p. 35.
206. Jāḥiẓ, *Ḥayawān*, III, pp. 131f.; ʿUsfūr, *Ṣūra*, p. 255.
207. Ibn Sīnā, *Shiʿr,* p. 174
208. "La théorie artistique la mieux élaborée au moyen âge est certainement la

théorie littéraire." De Bruyne, p. 243.
209. Nicholson, *Literary History*, pp. 329f.
210. Grabar, *Maqamat*.
211. Fahmī Muḥammad, "*Adab al-maqama*."
212. Bencheikh, *Poétique,* pp. 82f.
213. Abu Deeb, "Criticism," p. 368.
214. Lunde & Stone, p. 427.
215. Nicholson, *Literary History*, p. 309.
216. Abu Deeb, "Criticism," pp. 348ff.
217. Jurjānī, pp. 74, 147.
218. Heinrichs, *Dichtung*, pp. 54f.
219. Ibn Ṭabāṭabā, cited by Abu Deeb, "Criticism," p. 369.
220. Ayyad, p. 415.
221. ʿUṣfūr, *Qirāʾa,* pp. 155ff.; Schoeler, p. 116.
222. Bencheikh, *Poétique*, pp. 56ff. Ibn Khaldūn on poetry, *Muqaddima*, pp. 630–51.
223. Hamori, "Medieval Readers."
224. Ibn Khaldūn, *Muqaddima,* p. 636.
225. Von Grunebaum, *Kritik*, pp. 146f.
226. Nicholson, *Literary History*, p. 311.
227. Abu Deeb, *Jurjani*, pp. 275f.; Jurjānī, pp. 113f.
228. Heinrichs, *Dichtung*, pp. 69–99; Abu Deeb, "Criticism," p. 383.
229. Sperl, p. 27.
230. De Bruyne, p. 7.
231. Heinrichs, *Dichtung*, pp. 62f.
232. Sperl, pp. 168f.
233. "Le poème est le lieu de retrouvailles entre l'auditeur et le créateur." Bencheikh, *Poétique,* p. 145.
234. Jurjānī, p. 134; Abu Deeb, *Jurjani*, p. 276.
235. Khalafallah, "Badīʿ", *E.I.*[2]
236. Heinrichs, "Sariqa."
237. Grassi, pp. 169f.
238. ʿUṣfūr, *Ṣūra,* p. 326.
239. ʿUsfur, *Ṣūra,* p. 24.
240. Goodman, pp. 219f.
241. Arberry, *Aspects*, p. 132.
242. Eco, pp. 163f.
243. Eco, p. 166.
244. Ikhwān al-Ṣafā, III, p. 416.
245. Ikhwān al-Ṣafā, III, p. 420.
246. Dayihat translates the word *fikrī* with ratiocinatively [sic], p. 62.
247. Dahiyat, p. 63.
248. Goodman, pp. 219f.
249. ʿUṣfūr, *Ṣūra,* p. 190.
250. Abu Deeb, "Criticism," pp. 358ff., and *Jurjani*, pp. 136, 261; Jurjānī, p. 134.
251. Jurjānī, pp. 141ff.

252. ʿUṣfūr, *Ṣūra,* pp. 298, 302, 381.
253. Panofsky, p. 67; Pochat, p. 176.
254. Eco, pp. 172f., 175.
255. Fakhry, pp. 145f.
256. Fakhry, pp. 142ff; ʿUṣfūr, *Ṣūra*, pp. 28ff.; Goodman, pp. 146f.
257. Goichon, *Directives*, pp. 45, 507, 522.
258. Grassi, p.127.
259. Clevenot, p. 75.
260. Ibn Khaldūn, *Muqaddima,* pp. 449, 477, 589.
261. Ibn Khaldūn, *Muqaddima*, pp. 533f.
262. Ibn Khaldūn, *Muqaddima*, pp. 477ff., 526, 568ff.; Fakhry, pp. 326f.
263. Hawi, p. 164.
264. Rosenthal, *Knowledge*, p. 241.
265. Abū Ḥayyān, *Muqābasāt*, p. 60.
266. Abū Ḥayyān, *Imtāʿ*, II, p. 39; *Muqābasāt*, p. 292.
267. Abū Ḥayyān, *Muqābasāt*, pp. 101f.
268. Panofsky, p. 13.
269. Maqrīzī, II, p. 318; Ettinghausen, *Realism in Islamic Art.*
270. Ikhwān al-Ṣafā, I, p. 289.
271. Arberry, *Aspects*, p. 136; ʿUṣfūr, *Ṣūra,* p. 284.
272. Abu Deeb, *Jurjani*, pp. 264f. (with corrections); Jurjānī, p. 310.
273. Arkoun, *Essais*, p. 211.
274. Rebstock, pp. 55f.
275. Rebstock, pp. 82, 156; Necipoğlu, pp. 133, 139.
276. Galston, p. 144.
277. Galston, pp. 127ff., 141.
278. Arkoun, *Essais*, p. 267.
279. Ikhwān al-Ṣafā, I, p. 290.
280. De Bruyne, p. 42.
281. Ikhwān al-Ṣafā, I, pp. 284ff.
282. Ibn Khaldūn, *Muqaddima*, pp. 476–84.
283. Ibn Khaldūn, *Muqaddima*, p. 33.
284. Raymond, I, p. 215; Goitein, I, pp. 99, 106.
285. Biruni, *Gärten*, p. 215.
286. Rāghib al-Iṣfahānī, p. 203.
287. Maqrīzī, II, p. 318.
288. Behrens-Abouseif, "Building Craft."
289. Littmann, VI, 2, p. 454.
290. al-Shams, pp. 91f.
291. al-Shams, p. 93.
292. Clevenot, pp. 74f.
293. Farābī, *Iḥṣaʾ*, p. 34; Rosenthal, *Fortleben*, p. 94.
294. Ibn Khaldūn, *Muqaddima*, pp. 450ff.
295. Abu Ḥayyān, *Muqābasāt*, p. 312.
296. Bürgel, p. 99.
297. Maqrīzī, II, p. 183.

298. Maqrīzī, II, p. 382.
299. Maqrīzī, II, p. 316.
300. Kawkabānī, p. 42.
301. Maqrīzī, I, p. 32, II, pp. 101, 105.
302. Varisco, p. 8.
303. Behrens-Abouseif, "Physician."
304. Cf. Necipoğlu, pp. 133, 138.
305. Le Goff, p. 219; Castelnuovo, pp. 258f.
306. Behrens-Abouseif, "Building Craft."
307. Ettinghausen, "Decorative Art," p. 285; *Collected Papers*, p. 33.
308. Sourdel-Thomime, "Fann," *E.I.*[2]
309. Kroll, p. 153.
310. al-Maʿarrī, p. 518.
311. Cited by Sawa, p. 72.
312. Ibn al-Ḥājj, vol. 4, p. 198.
313. Creswell & Allan, p. 4.
314. Ibn Sīrīn (attr.), pp. 16, 224; Ibn Shāhīn, I, p. 311, II, 247.
315. Bosch, p. 6.
316. Ibn Qayyim, *Rawḍa*, p. 260.
317. Zarkashī, p. 336.
318. Ghazālī, III, p. 380.
319. Ibn Abī Zarʿ, p. 38.
320. Published by M. Amīn, *Tadhkira,* Appendix, p. 355.
321. Published by L. Mostafa, pp. 46ff.
322. al-Janab, p. 163.
323. Gabrieli & Scerrato, p. 305.
324. Amari, pp. 295, 298, 300, 303.
325. Ettinghausen & Grabar, p. 151.
326. Bourouiba, p. 63.
327. Hodgson, II, pp. 507ff.
328. Ettinghausen, "Hilāl," *E.I.*[2]
329. See Brend's comments on symbolism in her *Islamic Art*, pp. 226f.
330. Grabar, *Jerusalem*; Behrens-Abouseif, "Baptistère"; Leisten, "Mashhad al-Nasr."
331. Busse, "Fürstenspiegel."
332. Farès, p. 25.
333. Littmann, III, 2, "Die Geschichte von dem Streit über die Vorzüge der Geschlechter," pp. 579ff.
334. Behrens-Abouseif, "Baptistère."
335. Quoted by Arnold, p. 88.
336. Kawkabānī, pp. 40ff., trans. Arnold, p. 88; see also Rosenthal, *Fortleben*, p. 357, and Bosch et al., p. 10.
337. Ibn Ḥazm, p. 21.
338. Maqrīzī, II, p. 273.
339. Allen, *Essays*, p. 30.
340. Welch, p. 22.

341. Welch, p. 33.
342. Schimmel, p. 35.
343. Qalqashandī, III, pp. 20f.
344. Minorsky, p. 52.
345. Sabra, II, p. 303.
346. Rosenthal, "Penmanship," pp. 40f.
347. Biruni, *Gärten*, p. 215.
348. Safadi, pp. 11f.
349. Heinrichs, *Dichtung*, pp. 257f.
350. Shiloah, pp. 202f.
351. Abu Deeb, *Jurjani*, p. 316.
352. al-Faruqi, "Ornamentation," p. 18.
353. Kühnel, *Die Arabeske*.
354. Ettinghausen & Grabar, p. 151.
355. Grabar, *Alhambra*, p. 137; Maqrīzī, pp. 130–139.
356. De Bruyne, pp. 168, 214.
357. Marçais, *Esthétique*.
358. Ibn Khaldūn, *Muqaddima*, pp. 184–202, 325ff., 410ff.
359. Busse. "Fürstenspiegel," p. 161f.
360. Runciman, I, pp. 116f.
361. Maqrīzī, I, pp. 414ff.
362. Masʿūdī, II, p. 602.
363. Ibn Iyās, IV, p. 252.
364. Golombek, p. 32.
365. Ettinghausen & Hartner, "Conquering Lion."
366. Grabar, "What makes Islamic Art Islamic?" p. 2.
367. Serauky, p. 71.
368. Ibid.
369. Shirbīnī, p. 7.
370. Ibn Iyās, III, p. 240.
371. Maqrīzī, II, p. 318.
372. Grassi, pp. 127, 184.
373. Assunto, p. 22; De Bruyne, p. 228.
374. ʿAbd al-Wahhāb, p. 116.
375. Assunto, p.79.
376. Masʿūdī, II, p.434.
377. Nizāmulmulk, p. 162.
378. Ibn Khaldūn, *Muqaddima*, pp. 242f.
379. al-ʿAbbāsī, p. 165.
380. Cited by Creswell & Allan, p. 20.
381. Maqrīzī, II, p. 69.
382. Ibn Khaldūn, *Muqaddima,* pp. 450f.
383. Ibn Khaldūn, *Muqaddima*, pp. 32, 163.
384. Ibn Shāhīn, I, pp. 108f.
385. Ibn Abī Zarʿ, p. 59.
386. ʿAbd al-Wahhāb, p. 125.

387. Ibn Khaldūn, *Muqaddima*, p. 394.
388. Mujīr al-Dīn, II, p. 25.
389. Maqrīzī, II, p. 444.
390. Khalidi, *Masʿūdi*, p. 75.
391. Haarmann, p. 19 (Arabic text).
392. *Timur and the Princely Vision,* p. 43
393. Maqrīzī, II, p. 328.
394. Ibn Iyās, III, p. 413.
395. Haarmann, p. 47.
396. Cited by Creswell as epigraph to his book *Early Muslim Architecture.*
397. Ibn Khaldūn, *Muqaddima,* pp. 195.
398. De Sacy, pp. 186–96.
399. Maqrīzī, I, p. 120.
400. Jāhiẓ (attr.), *Maḥāsin*, pp. 1ff.; Bosch, pp. 5f.
401. ʿAzzām, II, p. 81.
402. al-Rashīd, p. 19.
403. Maqrīzī, II, p. 382.
404. Sakhāwī, II, p. 24.
405. Masʿūdī, II, p. 381.
406. Iṣbahānī, II, pp. 351f.
407. Ibn Iyās, V, p. 58.
408. The minaret of Aqbughā at the Azhar mosque. Maqrīzī, II, p. 384.

Bibliography

Literature in European Languages

Abu Deeb, K. *Al-Jurjānī's Theory of Poetic Imagery*. London, 1979.

Abu Deeb, K. "Literary Criticism." In *The Cambridge History of Arabic Literature. ʿAbbasid Belles-Lettres,* pp. 339–87.

ʿAbd al-Laṭīf al-Baghdādī: see de Sacy.

Affifi, A. E. *The Mystical Philosophy of Muḥyid Din Ibnul Arabi*. Cambridge, 1939.

Allen, T. *Five Essays on Islamic Art*. Sebastopol, Calif., 1988.

Allen, T. *Imagining Paradise in Islamic Art*. Sebastopol, Calif., 1993.

Amari, M. *Le Epigrafi Arabiche di Sicilia*, ed. F. Gabrieli. Palermo, 1971.

Arabian Nights (based on the text edited by Muhsin Mahdi), trans. Husain Haddawy. New York/London, 1990.

Arazi, A. "al-Shayb wa 'l-shabāb." *E.I.*[2]

Arberry, A. J. *Avicenna on Theology*. London, 1951.

Arberry, A. J. *The Poem of the Way*. London, 1952.

Arberry, A. J. *Revelation and Reason in Islam*. London, 1957.

Arberry, A. J. *Aspects of Islamic Civilization*. Ann Arbor, 1967.

Arkoun, M. *Traité d'Ethique*. Damascus, 1969.

Arkoun, M. *Essais sur la Pensée Islamique*. Paris, 1973.

Arkoun, M. "Islamic Culture, Modernity, Architecture." In *Architecture Education in the Islamic World* (Aga Khan Award for Architecture), 1986.

Arnaldez, R. "Ibn Ḥazm." *E.I.*[2]

Arnaldez, R. "Maʿrifa." *E.I.*[2]

Arnold, T. W. *Painting in Islam*. New York, 1965.

Assunto, R. *Die Theorie des Schönen im Mittelalter*. Köln, 1987.

Atıl, E. *Renaissance of Islam. Art of the Mamluks*. Washington, D.C., 1981.

Atıl, E., ed. *Islamic Art and Patronage*. New York, 1990.

Ayyad, S. M. "Regional Literature: Egypt." In *Cambridge History of Arabic Literature. ʿAbbasid Belles-Lettres*, pp. 412–41.

Behrens-Abouseif, D. "The Image of the Physician in Arab Biographies of the Post-Classical Period." *Der Islam* 66 (1989), pp. 331–43.

Behrens-Abouseif, D. "The Gardens of Islamic Egypt." *Der Islam* 69/2 (1992), pp. 76–82.

Behrens-Abouseif, D. "*Shād, Muhandis* and *Muʿallim*—Note on the Building Craft in the Mamluk Period." *Der Islam* 72/2 (1995), pp. 293–309.

Bencheikh, J. E. "Khamriyya." *E.I.*[2]

Bencheikh, J. E. *Poétique Arabe. Essai sur les Voies d'une Création*. Paris, 1975.

Berque, J. *Musiques sur le Fleuve. Les plus belles pages du kitâb al-aghâni.*

Paris, 1995.
al-Biruni. *In den Gärten der Wissenschaft*, trans. G. Strohmaier. Leipzig, 1991.
Blachère, R. *Histoire de la Littérature Arabe*. 3 vols. Paris, 1952–66.
Bosch, G., J. Carswell, and G. Petherbridge. *Islamic Bindings & Bookmaking*. Chicago, 1981.
Bosworth, C.E. *The Mediaeval Underworld, The Banū Sāsān in Arabic Society and Literature*. 2 vols. Leiden, 1976.
Bourouiba, R. *Les Inscriptions Commémoratives des Mosquées d'Algérie*. Algiers, 1977.
Brend, B. *Islamic Art*. Cambridge, Mass., 1991.
Brocchieri, M. F. B. "L'Intellectuel." In *L'Homme Médiéval.*, ed. J. Le Goff, pp. 225–32. Paris, 1987.
Brockelmann, C., and J. Vernet. "Al-Anṭākī." *E.I.*[2]
Bürgel, J. Ch. *The Feather of Simurgh. The "licit magic" of the Arts in Medieval Islam*. New York/London, 1988.
Bürgel, J. Ch. *Allmacht und Mächtigkeit. Religion und Welt im Islam*. Munich, 1991.
Burckhardt, T. *Art of Islam, Language and Meaning*. London, 1976.
Busse, H. "Fürstenspiegel und Fürstenethik im Islam." *Bustan* 1 (1968), pp. 12–19.
Butterworth, C. E., trans. & comment. *Averroes' Middle Commentary on Aristotle's Poetics*. Princeton, 1986.
Butterworth, C. E., ed. *The Political Aspects of Islamic Philosophy. Essays in Honor of Muhsin S. Mahdi*. Cambridge, Mass., 1992.
Calasso, G. "Les Remparts et la Loi, les Talismans et les Saints." *Bulletin d'Etudes Orientales* (Sciences Occultes et Islam) 44 (1992), pp. 83–104.
The Cambridge History of Arabic Literature ʿAbbasid Belles-Lettres, ed. J. Ashtiany and T. M. Johnstone. Cambridge, 1990.
Castelnuovo, E. "l'Artiste." In *L'Homme Médiéval*, ed. Le Goff, pp. 233–66. Paris, 1987.
Chebel, M. *Die Welt der Liebe im Islam—eine Enzyklopädie*. Munich, 1997.
Clevenot, D. *Une Esthétique du Voile*. Paris, 1994.
Corbin, H. *Suhrawardī d'Alep (+1191), Fondateur de la Doctrine Illuminative (ishrāqī)*. Paris, 1939.
Corbin, H. *Avicenne et le Récit Visionnaire*. 2 vols. Paris/Teheran, 1954.
Corbin, H. *L'Imagination Créatrice dans le Soufisme d'Ibn ʿArabi*. Paris, 1958.
Corbin, H. *Histoire de la Philosophie Arabe*. Paris, 1964.
Creswell, K. A. C. *The Muslim Architecture of Egypt*. 2 vols. Oxford, 1959.
Creswell, K. A. C. *Early Muslim Architecture*. 2 vols. Oxford, 1969.
Creswell, K. A. C., and J. Allan. *A Short Account of Early Muslim Architecture*. Aldershot, 1989.
Dahiyat, I. M. *Avicenna's Commentary on the Poetics of Aristotle*. Leiden, 1974.
Davidson, H. *Alfarabi, Avicenna and Averroes, on Intellect*. Oxford, 1992.
De Bruyne, *L'Esthétique du Moyen Age*. Louvain, 1947.
D'Erlanger, Baron R. *La Musique Arabe*. Vol. 4. Paris, 1939.
De Sacy, S. *Relation de l'Egypte par Abd-Allatif Médecin Arabe de Baghdad*.

Paris, 1810.

Dodd, C. E., and S. Khairallah. *The Image of the Word. A Study of Quranic Verses in Islamic Architecture*. Beirut, 1981.

Dols, M. W. *The Black Death in the Middle East*. Princeton, 1977.

Dubler, C. E. "Das Weiterleben der Antike im Islam." In *Das Erbe der Antike*, ed. F. Wehrli. Zürich/Stuttgart, 1963.

Duri, A. A. "Baghdād." *E.I.*[2]

During, J. "Le Grincement de la Porte du Paradis. La Double Structure de Phénomène Musical dans la Culture Islamique." In *Gott ist schön*, ed. A. Giese and Ch. Bürgel, pp. 153–75.

During, J. *Musique et Extase. L'Audition Mystique dans la Tradition Soufie*. Paris, 1988.

Eco, U. *Kunst und Schönheit im Mittelalter*. Munich/Vienna, 1991.

Ecochard, M. *Filiations des Monument Grecs, Byzantins et Islamiques*. Paris, 1977.

Elisseeff, N. *Thèmes et Motifs des Mille et Une Nuits*. Beirut, 1949.

Encyclopaedia of Islam. 2nd ed. (*E.I.*[2]) Leiden, 1968–.

Ettinghausen, R. "Ghazzāli on Beauty." In *Art and Thought, Issued in Honor of Dr. Ananda K. Coomaraswamy on the Occasion of His 70th Birthday*, ed. K. Bharatna Iyer, pp. 160–65. London/Luzac, 1947. Repr. in *Islamic Art and Archaeology. Collected Papers*, pp. 16–21.

Ettinghausen, R. "Early Realism in Islamic Art." *Studi Orientalistici in Onore di Giorgio Levi Della Vida*. Vol. 1, pp. 250–73. Rome, 1956. Repr. in *Islamic Art and Archaeology. Collected Papers*, pp. 158–81.

Ettinghausen, R., and W. Hartner. "The Conquering Lion, the Life and Cycle of a Symbol." *Oriens* 17 (1964), pp. 161–71. Repr. in *Islamic Art and Archaeology. Collected Papers*, pp. 693–712.

Ettinghausen, R. "Decorative Art and Painting: Their Character and Scope." In *Legacy of Islam*, ed. J. Schacht and C. E. Bosworth, pp. 274–92. Oxford, 1974. Repr. in *Islamic Art and Archaeology. Collected Papers*, pp. 22–50.

Ettinghausen, R. "Originality and Conformity in Islamic Art," repr. in *Islamic Art and Archaeology. Collected Papers*, pp. 89–156.

Ettinghausen, R. *Islamic Art and Archaeology. Collected Papers*, ed. M. Rosen-Ayalon. Berlin, 1976.

Ettinghausen, R., and O. Grabar. *The Art and Architecture of Islam (650–1250)*. New York, 1987.

Fahd, T. *La Divination Arabe, Etudes Religieuses, Sociologiques, et Folkloriques sur le Milieu Natif de l'Islam*. Leiden, 1966.

Fakhry, M. *A History of Islamic Philosophy*. London/New York, 1983.

Farès, B. *Essai sur l'Esprit de la Décoration Islamique*. Cairo, 1952.

Farmer, H. G. "The Influence of Music: from Arabic Sources." *Proceedings of the Musical Association* 52 (1925–26), pp. 89–124. Repr. in Farmer, *Studies in Oriental Music*, vol. 1, pp. 291–328.

Farmer, H. G. *"Music: the Priceless Jewel. From the Kitab al-ʿIqd al-Farīd of Ibn ʿAbd Rabbihi (d. 949) Edited and Translated*. Published by the Author, Bearsden, 1942.

Farmer, H. G. "Al-Kindī on Ethos of Rhythm, Colour, and Perfume." *Transactions of the Glasgow University Oriental Society* 17 (1955–56), pp. 29–38.

Farmer, H. G. *A History of Arabian Music to the XIIth Century*. London, 1967.

Farmer, H. G. *Studies in Oriental Music* (reprint of publications from the years 1925–66), ed. E. Neubauer. 2 vols. Frankfurt, 1986.

al-Faruqi, L. I. "Ornamentation in Arabian Improvisational Music: A Study of Interrelatedness in the Arts." *World of Music* 1 (1978), pp. 17–28.

al-Faruqi, L. I. *The Nature of the Musical Art of Islamic Culture: A Theoretical and Empirical Study of Arabian Music*. Ph.D. diss., Syracuse University, New York, 1964.

Gabrieli, F., and U. Scerrato. *Gli Arabi in Italia*. Milano, 1989.

Gabrieli, G. "Adab." *E.I.*[2]

Galston, M. "The Theoretical and Practical Dimensions of Happiness as Portrayed in the Political Treatises of al-Farābī." In Butterworth, *Political Aspects*, pp. 95–151.

Gardet, L. *La Pensée Religieuse d'Avicenne*. Paris, 1951.

Gardet, L. "D̲janna." *E.I.*[2]

Gardet, L., and Anawati, G. C. *Mystique Musulmane: Aspects et Tendances, Expériences et Techniques*. Paris, 1961.

Gardet, L. *Les Grands Problèmes de la Théologie Musulmane: Dieu et la Destinée de l'Homme*. Paris, 1967.

Gaudefroy-Demombynes. *Ibn Qotaiba. Introduction au Livre de la Poésie et des Poètes*. Paris, 1947.

The Genius of Arab Civilization. Source of Renaissance. Cambridge, Mass., 1975.

Geries, I. *Un Genre Littéraire Arabe: al-Maḥāsin wa 'l-Masāwī*. Paris, 1977.

Ghazālī, Abū Ḥāmid Muḥammad. *The Alchemy of Happiness*, trans. C. Field and E. Daniel. New York/London, 1991.

Ghazi, M.F. "Un groupe social: 'Les Raffinés' (ẓurafāʾ)." *Studia Islamica* 11 (1959), pp. 39–71.

Giese, A., and Ch. Bürgel, eds. *Gott ist schön und Er liebt die Schönheit. Festschrift für Annemarie Schimmel*. Bern, 1992.

Goichon, A.-M., trans. *Ibn Sīnā. Livre des Directives et Remarques (kitāb al-ishārāt wa l-tanbīhāt)*. Paris, 1951.

Goichon, A.-M. "Ḥayy b. Yaqẓān." *E.I.*[2]

Goichon, A.-M. "Ibn Sīnā." *E.I.*[2]

Goitein, S. D. *A Mediterranean Society*. Vol. 1, *Economic Foundations*. Berkeley, 1967.

Goldziher, I. *A Short History of Classical Arabic Literature*. Trans. & rev. J. Desomogyi. Hildesheim, 1966.

Golombek, L. "The Draped Universe of Islam." In *Content and Context of Visual Arts in the Islamic World*, ed. P. Soucek. London, 1988.

Gombrich, *The Sense of Order*. London, 1994.

Goodmann, L. E. *Avicenna*. London/New York, 1992.

Grabar, O. "The Earliest Islamic Commemorative Structures Notes and

Documents." *Ars Orientalis* 6 (1966), pp. 7–46.
Grabar, O. "Imperial and Urban Art in Islam." In *Colloque International sur l'Histoire du Caire 27 Mars–5 Avril 1969*, pp. 173–190. Cairo, 1969.
Grabar, O. "What Makes Islamic Art Islamic." *AARP* (*Art and Archaeology Research Papers*), April 1976, pp. 1–3.
Grabar, O. *Die Alhambra*. Köln, 1981.
Grabar, O. *The Illustrations of the Maqāmāt*. Chicago/London, 1984.
Grabar, O. "The Iconography of Islamic Architecture." In *Content and Context of Visual Arts in the Islamic World*, ed. P. Soucek, pp. 51–60. London, 1988.
Grabar, O. "Patronage in Islamic Art." In *Islamic Art and Patronage. Treasures from Kuwayt*, ed. Esin Atil, pp. 27–39. New York, 1990.
Grabar, O. *The Mediation of Ornament*. Princeton, 1992.
Grabar, O. *The Shape of the Holy. Early Islamic Jerusalem*. Princeton, 1996.
Green, A. H., ed. *In Quest of an Islamic Humanism*. Cairo, 1984.
Guthrie, S. *Arab Social Life in the Middle Ages*. London, 1995.
Grassi, E. *Die Theorie des Schönen in der Antike*. Köln, 1980.
Grunebaum, G. von. *Kritik und Dichtkunst. Studien zur arabischen Literaturgeschichte*. Wiesbaden, 1955.
Grünert, M. *Der Löwe in der Literatur der Araber*. Prague, 1899.
Haarmann, U. *Das Pyramidenbuch des Abū Ǧaʿfar al-Idrīsī*. Beirut, 1991.
Hamori, A. *On the Art of Medieval Arabic Literature*. Princeton, 1974.
Hamori, A. "Did Medieval Readers Make Sense of Form? Notes on a Passage from al-Iskāfī." In *In Quest of an Islamic Humanism*, ed. A.H. Green, pp. 39–47. Cairo, 1984.
Hawi, S. *Islamic Naturalism and Mysticism*. Leiden, 1974.
Heine, P. *Weinstudien: Untersuchungen zum Anbau, Produktion und Konsum des Weins im arabisch-islamischen Mittelalter*. Wiesbaden, 1982.
Heine, P. *Kulinarische Studien. Untersuchungen zur Kochkunst im arabisch-islamischen Mittelalter*. Wiesbaden, 1988.
Heinrichs, W. *Arabische Dichtung und Griechische Poetik*. Beirut, 1969.
Heinrichs, W. "An Evaluation of Sariqa." *Quaderni dei Studi Arabe* 5–6 (1987–88), pp. 357–68.
Herzfeld, E. *Der Wandschmuck der Bauten von Samarra und seine Ornamentik*. Berlin, 1923.
Hill, D. *Islamic Science and Engineering*. Edinburgh, 1993.
Hillenbrand, C. "Some Aspects of al-Ghazālī's Views on Beauty." In *Gott ist schön*, ed. Giese and Bürgel, pp. 249–265.
Hillenbrand, R. "La Dolce Vita in Early Islamic Syria of Later Umayyad Palaces." *Art History* 5 (1987), pp. 1–35.
Hodgson, M. G. S. *The Venture of Islam*. Vol. 2. Chicago, 1964.
Horovitz, J. "Die Beschreibung eines Gemäldes bei Mutanabbī." *Der Islam* 1 (1910), pp. 385–89.
Holod, R. "Plan and Building: On the Transmission of Architectural Knowledge." In *Theories and Principles of Design in the Architecture of Islamic Societies*. Cambridge, Mass., 1988.
Homerin, E. *From Arab Poet to Muslim Saint*. Columbia, S.C., 1994.

Hourani, G. "The Principal Subject of Ibn Ṭufayl's Ḥayy Ibn Yaqzān." *Journal of the Near-Eastern Studies* 15 (1956), pp. 40–46.
James, D. *Qur'ans of the Mamluks*. London, 1988.
al-Janab, T. J. *Studies in Mediaeval Iraqi Architecture*. Baghdad, 1983.
Kahwaji, S. "ʿIlm al-Djamāl." *E.I.*[2]
Khairallah, A. E. *Love, Madness, and Poetry. An Interpretation of the Mağnūn Legend*. Beirut, 1980.
Khalafallah, M. "Badīʿ." *E.I.*[2]
Khalidi, T. *Islamic Historiography. The Histories of Masʿūdi*. Albany, 1975.
Khalidi, T. *Arabic Historical Thought in the Classical Period*. Cambridge, 1996.
Kraemer, J. L. *Humanism in the Renaissance of Islam. The Cultural Revival During the Buyid Age*. Leiden, 1986.
Kroll, F.-L. *Das Ornament in der Kunsttheorie des 19. Jahrhunderts*. Zürich/New York, 1987.
Kuehnel, E. *Die Arabeske*. Wiesbaden, 1949.
Le Goff, J., ed. *L'Homme Médiéval*. Paris, 1987.
Le Goff, J. *La Civilisation de l'Occident Médiéval*. Paris, 1988.
Leisten, T. "Mashhad al-Nasr: Monuments of War and Victory in Medieval Islam," *Muqarnas* 13 (1996), pp. 7–26.
Lewis, B. "Siyāsa." In *In Quest of an Islamic Humanism*, ed. A. H. Green, pp. 3–14. Cairo, 1984.
Lings, M., and Y. H. Safadi. *The Qur'an*. A British Library Exhibition. World of Islam Festival, 1976.
Littmann, E. *Die Erzählungen aus den Tausendundein Nächten*. 6 vols. Frankfurt, 1981.
Lunde, P., and C. Stone, trans. and ed. *The Meadows of Gold. The Abbasids*. London/New York, 1989.
Mahdi, M. *Alfarabi's Philosophy of Plato and Aristotle*. New York, 1962.
Mahdi, M. "Islamic Philosophy and the Fine Arts." In *Architecture and Community. Building in the Islamic World Today* (Aga Khan Award for Architecture), 1983.
El-Mallah, I. *Arab Music and Musical Notation*. Tutzing, 1997.
Marçais, G. "Remarques sur l'Esthétique Musulmane." *Annales de l'Institut d'Etudes Orientales*, Tome 4 (1938), pp. 55–71.
Marçais, G. "Nouvelles Remarques sur l'Esthétique Musulmane," *Annales de l'Institut d'Etudes Orientales*, Tome 6 (1942–47), pp. 31–71.
Marçais, G. *L'Architecture Musulmane d'Occident*. Paris, 1954.
Massignon, L. *La Passion d'al-Ḥallāj*. Paris, 1922.
Mehren, A. F. *Die Rhetorik der Araber*. Copenhagen and Vienna, 1853.
Meinecke, M. *Die Mamlukische Architektur in Ägypten und Syrien*. 2 vols. Glückstadt, 1992.
Mez, A. *Die Renaissance des Islams*. 2 vols. Heidelberg, 1922.
Minorsky, V., trans. *Calligraphers and Painters. A treatise by Qāḍī Aḥmad son of Mīr Munshī*. Washington, 1959.
Miquel, A. *Sept Contes des Mille et Une Nuits*. Paris, 1987.
Mostafa, S. L. (and F. Jaritz). "Madrasa, Ḫānqāh und Mausoleum des Barqūq in

Kairo." *Abhandlungen des Deutschen Archäologischen Instituts Kairo* 4 (1982), pp. 36–139.

Müller, H. *Die Kunst des Sklavenkaufs*. Freiburg, 1980.

Naff, T. "History and Reform in Islam." In *In Quest of an Islamic Humanism*, ed. A. H. Green, pp. 123–38. Cairo, 1984.

Nasr, S. H. *An Introduction to Islamic Cosmological Doctrines*. London, 1964.

Nassar, N. *La Pensée réaliste d'Ibn Khaldūn*. Paris, 1967.

Necipoğlu, G. *The Topkapı Scroll. Geometry and Ornament in Islamic Architecture*. Santa Monica, 1995.

Neubauer, E. *Musiker am Hofe der frühen Abbasiden*. Frankfurt a.M., 1965.

Nicholson, R. A. *A Literary History of the Arabs*. London, 1907; reprinted Cambridge, 1953, 1969.

Nicholson, R. A. *The Mystics of Islam*. London, 1989.

Nizāmulmulk, *Das Buch der Staatskunst Siyāsatnāma*, trans. K. E. Schabinger. Zürich, 1987.

O'Leary, D. *Arabic Thought and its Place in History*. London, 1939.

Panofsky, E. *Idea. Ein Beitrag zur Begriffsgeschichte der älteren Kunsttheorie*. Berlin, 1960.

Papadopoulo, A., ed. *Le Miḥrāb dans l'Architecture et la Religion Musulmanes*. Leiden/New York, 1988.

Pellat, Ch. *Arabische Geisteswelt Dargestellt von Charles Pellat auf Grund der Schriften von al-Ğāḥiẓ 777–869*. Zürich/Stuttgart, 1967.

Pellat, Ch. "Ḥikāya." *E.I.*[2]

Pellat, Ch. "Ḳayna." *E.I.*[2]

Pellat, Ch. "Maḳāma." *E.I.*[2]

Pandit, S. *An Approach to the Indian Theory of Art and Aesthetics*. New Delhi, 1977.

Pochat, G. *Geschichte der Ästhetik und Kunsttheorie—von der Antike bis zum 19. Jahrhundert*. Köln, 1986.

al-Qaddūmī, G., trans. & ed. *Book of Gifts and Rarities (Kitāb al-Hadāyā wa al-Tuḥaf)*. Cambridge, Mass., 1990.

al-Rashīd, S. *Darb Zubayda. The Pilgrim Road from Kufa to Mecca*. Riyadh, 1980.

Raymond, A. *Artisans et Commerçants au Caire au XVIIIe Siècle*. 2 vols. Damascus, 1973.

Rebstock, U. *Rechnen im islamischen Orient*. Darmstadt 1992.

Ritter, H., trans. *Al-Ghasāli. Das Elixier der Glückseligkeit*. Munich, 1989.

Rosenthal, F. "Abu Haiyan al-Tawḥīdī on Penmanship." *Ars Islamica* 13–14 (1948), pp. 1–30.

Rosenthal, F. *Das Fortleben der Antike im Islam*. Zürich/Stuttgart, 1965.

Rosenthal, F. *Knowledge Triumphant: The Concept of Knowledge in Medieval Islam*. Leiden, 1970.

Rosenthal, F. *Four Essays on Art and Literature in Islam*. Leiden, 1971.

Rückert, F. *Al-Harīrī. Die Verwandlungen des Abu Seid von Serug*, with an afterword by W. Walter. Leipzig, 1989.

Rückert, F. *Orientalische Dichtung*, ed. A-M. Schimmel. Bremen, 1963.

Runciman, S. *A History of the Crusades*. 2 vols. London, 1990.
Russell, G. A. "The Rusty Mirror of the Mind: Ibn Ṭufayl's and Ibn Sīnā's Psychology." In *The World of Ibn Ṭufayl: Interdisciplinary Perspectives on Ḥayy Ibn Yaqẓān*, ed. L. Conrad. Leiden, 1991.
Sabra, A.I. (trans. & comment.) *The Optics of Ibn al-Haytham. Books I–III On Direct Vision*. 2 vols. London, 1989.
Sadan, J., A.K. Reinhard, and B. Reinert, "Shaʿr." *E.I.*[2]
Safadi, Y. H. *Islamic Calligraphy*. New York, 1987.
el-Said, I., and A. Parman. *Geometric Concepts in Islamic Art*. London, 1976.
Sawa, G. D. *Music Performance Practice in the Early ʿAbbāsid Era*. Toronto, 1989.
Schatzmiller, M. *Labor in the Medieval Islamic World*. Leiden/New York/Köln, 1994.
Schimmel, A. *Calligraphy and Islamic Culture*. New York, 1984.
Schoeler, G. *Arabische Naturdichtung*. Beirut, 1974.
Sellheim, R. "Das Lächeln des Propheten," in *Festschrift für A. D. E. Jensen*, vol. 2, pp. 621–34. Munich, 1964.
Serauky, E. "Das Verhältnis zwischen Beduinen und Ansässigen im 9./10. Jh. in Zentralgebieten des islamischen Kalifats." In *Ibn Ḫaldūn und seine Zeit*, ed. D. Sturm, pp. 69–76. Halle, 1983.
Shehadi, F. *Philosophies of Music in Medieval Islam*. Leiden/New York/Köln, 1995.
Shiloah, A., trans. and ed. al-Kātib, al-Ḥasan Ibn Aḥmad Ibn ʿAli. *La Perfection des Connaissances Musicales (Kitāb kamāl adab al-ġināʾ)*. Paris, 1972.
Sourdel, D. and J. *La Civilisation de l'Islam Classique*. Paris, 1983.
Sperl, S. *Mannerism in Arabic Poetry—A Structural Analysis of Selected Texts (3d century AH/9th century AD–5th century AH/11th century AD)*. Cambridge/New York, 1989.
Tatarkiewicz, W. *History of Aesthetics*, ed. C. Barrett. 2 vols. The Hague/Paris, 1970.
Thackston, W. M., trans. *The Mystical and Visionary Treatises of Shihabuddin Yahya Suhrawardi*. London, 1982.
Timur and the Princely Vision. Persian Art and Culture in the Fifteenth Century. Los Angeles, 1989.
Trabulsi, A. *La Critique Poétique des Arabes*. Damascus, 1955.
Vadet, J. C. *L'Esprit Courtois en Orient dans les Cinq Premiers Siècles de l'Hégire*. Paris, 1968.
Van Gelder, G. J. *The Bad and the Ugly. Attitudes Towards Invective Poetry (Hijāʾ) in Classical Arabic Literature*. Leiden/New York, 1988.
Varisco, D. M. *Medieval Agriculture and Islamic Science*. Seattle/London, 1994.
Watt, W. M. *Islamic Philosophy and Theology*. Edinburgh, 1962.
Walzer, R. *Greek into Arabic: Essays on Islamic Philosophy*. Oxford, 1962.
Welch, A. *Calligraphy in the Arts of the Muslim World*. New York, 1979.
Wensinck, A. J. *La Pensée de Ghazzalī*. Paris, 1940.

Literature in Arabic

ʿAbbās, I. *Tārīkh al-naqd al-adabī ʿinda ʾl-ʿarab*. 2nd ed. Amman, 1993.

al-ʿAbbāsī, Ibn ʿAbd Allāh al-Ḥasan. *Āthār al-uwal fī tartīb al-duwal*. Cairo, 1295H.

ʿAbd al-Raḥmān, ʿA. *al-Ghufrān li- Abī ʾl-ʿAlāʾ al-Maʿarrī*. Cairo, 1962.

ʿAbd al-Wahhāb, Ḥ. "al-Rusūmāt al-handasiyya li'l-ʿimāra ʾl-islāmiyya." *Al-Muʾtamar al-Thānī li'l-Āthār fi-l-bilād al-ʿArabiyya*, pp. 107–29. Cairo, 1958.

Abū-Ḥayyān al-Tawḥīdī. *Thalāth rasāʾil*, ed. Ibrāhīm al-Kaylānī. Damascus, 1951.

Abū-Ḥayyān al-Tawḥīdī. *al-Imtāʿ waʾl-muʾānasa*. Beirut, 1953.

Abū-Ḥayyān al-Tawḥīdī. *al-Muqābasāt*. Beirut, 1989.

Abū Nuwās. *Dīwān*. Beirut, n.d.

Alf Laylā wa Laylā, ed. M. Mahdī. Leiden, 1984.

Amīn, B. Sh. *Muṭālaʿāt fī ʾl-shiʿr al-mamlūki wa ʾl-ʿuthmānī*. Beirut, 1979.

ʿAzzām,ʿA. *Majlis al-Sulṭān al-Ghūrī*. 2 vols. Cairo, 1941.

Badawī, ʿAbd al-Raḥmān. *Aflūṭīn ʿinda ʾl-ʿarab*. 3rd ed. Cairo, 1977.

Fahmī Muḥammad, ʿAbd al-Raḥman. "Bayn adab al-maqāma wa fann al-ʿimāra fī ʾl-madrasa al-saʿdiyya." *Majallat al-majmaʿ al-ʿilmī al-miṣrī* 52 (1970–71), pp. 39–63.

al-Farābī. *Iḥṣāʾ al-ʿulūm*, ed. ʿU. Amīn. Cairo, 1949.

al-Farābī. *Kitāb al-musīqī al-kabīr*, ed. Gh. Khashaba. Cairo, 1967.

al-Ghazālī. *Iḥyāʾ ʿulūm al-dīn*, 16 vols. Cairo, 1357/1938–39.

al-Ḥarīrī. *Sharḥ maqāmāt al-ḥarīrī*, with commentary by Ibn al-Khashshāb and Ibn Barbarī. n.p.: Dār al-Fikr, 1326/1908–9.

Ḥāzim al-Qarṭājannī. *Minhāj al-bulaghāʾ wa sarāj al-udabāʾ*, ed. M. H. Ibn al-Khūjā. Tunis, 1966.

Ḥilmī, M. K. *Abū ʾl-Ṭayyib al-Mutanabbī*. Damascus, 1986.

Ibn Abī Hajla. *Dīwān al-ṣabāba*. Cairo, 1279H.

Ibn Abī Zarʿ. *al-Anīs al-muṭrib bi rawḍ al-qirṭās*. Rabat, 1973.

Ibn Ḥabīb. *Tadhkirat al-nabīh fī ayyām al-manṣūr wa banīh*, ed. M. Amīn. Vol. 1. Cairo 1976.

Ibn al-Ḥājj. *al-Madkhal*. 4 vols. Beirut, 1981.

Ibn al-Haytham: see Sabra.

Ibn Ḥazm. *Ṭawq al-ḥamāma*. Beirut, 1992.

Ibn Iyās. *Badāʾiʿ al-zuhūr fi waqʾāiʿ al-duhūr*, ed. M. Muṣṭafā. 5 vols. Cairo, 1961–1975.

Ibn al-Kātib: see Shiloah.

Ibn Khaldūn. *Al-Muqaddima*. Beirut, n.d.

Ibn Khaldūn. *al-Taʿrīf bi Ibn Khaldūn*. Beirut, 1979.

Ibn Qayyim al-Jawziyya. *Rawḍat al-muḥibbīn*. Cairo, n.d.

Ibn Qayyim al-Jawziyya. *al-Ṭibb al-nabawī*. Cairo, n.d.

Ibn Qayyim al-Jawziyya. *Zād al-maʿād*. Cairo, 1324/1906–7.

Ibn Shāhīn, Khalīl. *Tafsīr al-aḥlām al-musammā al-isharāt fī ʿilm al-ʿibārāt*. 2 vols. Cairo, 1991.

Ibn Sīnā. *Fann al-shiʿr min kitāb al-shifāʾ*, ed. ʿA. Badawī. Cairo, 1953.

Ibn Sīnā: see Goichon, *Directives*.
Ibn Sīrīn, M. (attributed to). *Tafsīr al-aḥlām*. Beirut, 1995.
Ibn al-Zubayr. *Kitāb al-dhakhā'ir wa 'l-tuḥaf*, ed. M. Ḥamīd Allāh. Kuwayt, 1959.
al-Idrīsī: see Haarmann.
Ikhwān al-Ṣafā. *Rasā'il*. 4 vols. Beirut, n.d.
al-Iṣbahānī. *Kitāb al-aghānī*. 24 vols. Cairo, 1963.
Ismāʿīl, I. *al-Usūs al-jamāliyya fī 'l-naqd al-adabī*. Cairo, 1968.
al-Jāḥiz, Ibn ʿUthmān ʿUmar Ibn Baḥr. *al-Ḥayawān*, ed. ʿA. Hārūn and M. B. Ḥalabī. Cairo, 1948.
al-Jāḥiz (attributed to). *Al-Kitāb al-musammā bi'l-maḥāsin wa'l-aḍdād (Le Livre des Beautés et des Antithèses)*, ed. Gerlov Van Vloten. Leyden, 1898; repr. Amsterdam, 1974.
al-Jurjānī, ʿAbd al-Qāhir. *Asrār al-balāgha fī ʿilm al-bayān*. Beirut, 1995.
al-Jurjānī, al-Qāḍī ʿAbd al-ʿAzīz. *al-Wasāṭa bayna al-mutanabbī wa khuṣūmihi*, ed. Muḥ. Abu'l-Faḍl Ibrāhīm and Muḥ. al-Bajawī. Cairo, 1945.
al-Kātib, al-Ḥasan Ibn Aḥmad. *Kitāb kamāl adab al-ghinā*, ed. G. ʿA. Khashaba. Cairo, 1975. See also Shiloah.
al-Kawkabānī. *Ḥadā'iq al-nammām fī 'l-kalām ʿalā mā yataʿallaq bi'l-ḥammām*. Beirut, 1986.
Kurd ʿAlī, Muḥammad. *Rasā'il al-bulāghā'*. Cairo, 1954.
al-Maʿarrī, Abū 'l-ʿAlā. *Risālat al-Ghufrān*, ed. ʿA. ʿAbd al-Raḥmān. Cairo, 1963.
al-Maqrīzī. *al-Mawāʿiz wa'l-iʿtibār fī dhikr al-khiṭaṭ wa'l-āthār*. Būlāq, 1270/1853–4.
al-Masʿūdī. *Murūj al-dhahab*. 2 vols. Beirut, 1982.
Mujīr al-Dīn. *al-Uns al-jalīl bi tārīkh al-Quds wa'l-Khalīl*. 2 vols. Amman, 1973.
Mubārak, Z. *al-Taṣawwuf al-islāmī fī 'l-adab wa'l-akhlāq*. 2 vols. Cairo, n.d.
al-Nawājī. *Ḥulbat al-kumayt fī'l-adab wa 'l-nawādir al-mutaʿalliqa bi 'l-khamriyyāt*. Cairo 1299/1881–82.
al-Qalqashandī. *Subḥ al-aʿshā fī ṣināʿat al-inshā*. 14 vols. Cairo, 1963.
al-Rāghib al-Iṣfahānī. *al-Dharīʿa ʿalā makārim al-sharīʿa*, ed. Ṭ. ʿA. Saʿd. Cairo, 1973.
Saʿd, F. *Khayāl al-ẓill al-ʿarabī*. Beirut, 1993.
al-Sakhāwī, Shams al-Dīn Muḥ. *al-Ḍaw' al-lāmiʿ li-ahl al-qarn al-tāsiʿ*. 12 vols. Cairo, 1896.
Salīm, M. R. *ʿAṣr salāṭīn al-mamālīk wa nitājuhu 'l-ʿilmī wa'l-adabī*. 8 vols. Cairo, 1962.
al-Shāmī, A. *al-Ẓāhira al-Ẓamāliyya fī 'l-islām*. Beirut, 1986.
al-Shams, M. ʿAbd Allāh. *Muqaddima li ʿilm al-mīkānīk fī 'l-ḥaḍāra al-ʿarabiyya*. Vol. 1. Baghdad, 1977.
al-Shirbīnī. *Hazz al-quhūf fī sharḥ qaṣīd abī-shādūf*. Cairo, 1890–91.
al-Suhrawardī, Yaḥyā. *Ḥikmat al-ishrāq. Opera Metaphysica et Mystica*, ed. H. Corbin. Paris/Teheran, 1952.
ʿUṣfūr, J. *Qirā'at al-turāth al-naqdī*. Kuwait, 1992.
ʿUṣfūr, J. *al-Ṣūra 'l-fanniya fī 'l-turāth al-naqdī wa 'l-balāghī*. Cairo, 1992.
al-Washsha', Abū Ṭayyib Muḥammad Ibn Isḥāq. *Kitāb al-muwashshā*, ed. R.

Brünnow. Leiden, 1886.
al-Zabīdī, Muḥammad Murtaḍā. *Ḥikmat al-ishrāq ilā kuttāb al-āfāq*. Cairo, 1374/1954.
al-Zarkashī, Muḥammad Ibn ʿAbd Allāh. *Iʿlam al-sājid bi-aḥkām al-masājid*. Cairo, 1397/1976–77.
al-Zawzanī. *Sharḥ al-muʿallāqāt al-sabʿ*. Cairo, 1958.

*Biographical Notes**

Abū Ḥanīfa, al-Nuʿmān (born around 699 probably in Kufa, died in 767 in Baghdad), was the founder of the Ḥanafī school *(madhhab)* of Islamic law, named for him, which is one of the four acknowledged rites of Sunni Islam. Little is known about his life. His grandfather is said to have been a manumitted slave from Kabul. Abū Ḥanīfa himself did not write books on Islamic Law, but he communicated his ideas to his disciples and students through teaching, dictating, and discussions.

Abū Nuwās, Ḥasan (born between 747 and 762 in al-Ahwāz/Khuzistan in southern Iran, died between 813 and 815 in Baghdad), was the most famous Arab poet of the Abbasid period. His mother was Persian and his father of South Arabian origin. Abū Nuwās lived in Basra, Kufa, and finally in Baghdad; he is reported to have spent some time among bedouins in order to refine his knowledge of the Arabic language. He spent the most successful years of his career at the court of the Caliph Amīn, and also enjoyed the patronage of the Barmakīds (a dynasty of viziers at the Abbasid court). However, he faced serious problems because of the excessive libertinage expressed in his love and wine poetry. In traditional Arabic literary criticism Abū Nuwās is considered the foremost representative of the modernist school, as opposed to the pre-Islamic classical school. There are contradictory reports about his death, all typical of his character. He may have died in prison, convicted for blasphemy, or in a tavern, or in the house of a family of scholars and friends.

al-ʿ**Āmirī**, Abū 'l-Ḥasan Muḥammad (born in the early 10th century in Khorasan, died in 992 in Nishapur/Khorasan), was a philosopher of Neoplatonic and Aristotelian orientation who tried to reconcile philosophical with religious thought. He was sponsored by the viziers of the Buyid dynasty in Rayy. His two visits to Baghdad, where he was treated as an ill-mannered provincial, did not bring him success.

al-**Ashʿarī**, Abū 'l-Ḥasan ʿAlī (born 873/74 in Basra, died in 935/36 in Baghdad), was the founder of the theological school named after him. He began his career as Muʿtazilit (a rationalistic school of theology strongly influenced by Greek thought), but found the way back to orthodoxy in 912/13, apparently after having had a dream where the Prophet blamed him for his unorthodox belief.

al-**Aṣmaʿī**, Abū Saʿīd ʿAbd al-Malik (born in 740 and died around 828 in Basra), was a philologist and a literary critic. In order to refine his knowledge of the Arabic language he spent some time among bedouins. He attracted a large number of students in Basra and in Baghdad, where he was also hired by the

* Based on the *Encyclopaedia of Islam*, 2nd ed.

caliph Harūn al-Rashīd, whom he entertained with anecdotes.

al-**Bīrūnī**, Abū 'l-Rayḥān Muḥammad (born in 973 in Kāth/Khawarizm south of the Aral lake, died around 1048 probably in Ghazna). Combining the knowledge of a natural scientist, astronomer, historian, and geographer, he was one of the most outstanding scholars of the Islamic middle ages. His sponsors were the Samanid sultan Manṣūr II Ibn Nūḥ in Bukhara and the Ziyarid Abū 'l-Ḥasan Qābūs in Jurjān along the Caspian Sea, to whom he dedicated his first major work about chronology. He then went to the court of the Ghaznawid ruler Maḥmūd, where he compiled a major and exceptional book on India.

Dhū 'l-Nūn, Abū 'l-Fayḍ Thawbān (born in 796 in Ikhmīm/Upper Egypt, died in Gizah), was one of the earliest sufis and the first to teach sufism systematically as a doctrine. His father was Nubian and he himself perhaps a manumitted slave. He traveled to Mecca, Damascus, and Antioch. Facing the hostility of the rationalist Muʿtazilits as well as of the Orthodox, he was sent to jail, but was set free by order of the Abbasid caliph. In the Islamic guild literature Dhū 'l-Nūn is the patron saint of physicians.

al-**Fārābī**, Abū Naṣr Muḥammad (born in 870 in Fārāb in Transoxiana, died in 950 in Damascus). Known in Latin texts as Alfarabius or Avennasar, he was one of the greatest Muslim philosophers and musicologists. His father was most likely a Turkish officer in the personal guard of the caliph in Baghdad. Sayf al-Dawla, the Hamdanid ruler of Aleppo, invited him to his court where he had surrounded himself with scholars. Al-Farābī sought to reconcile Plato's thought with Aristotle's in an Islamic Neoplatonism.

al-**Ghazālī**, Abū Ḥāmid Muḥammad (born in 1058 in Ṭūs/Khorasan, died in 1111 in Ṭus) was one of the foremost theologians and reformers of Islam. He taught in Baghdad at the famous *madrasa* of Niẓām al-Mulk and withdrew as a sufi and private scholar to Damascus before returning to Ṭūs. During this period he wrote his most famous book *Iḥyāʾ ʿUlūm al-Ḍīn* ("The revival of the religious sciences"). His great contribution to Islam was to integrate sufism into orthodoxy.

Ibn ʿArabī, Muḥyī al-Dīn Muḥammad (born in 1165 in Murcia, died in 1240 in Damascus), was one of the greatest sufis of Islam and the most prolific writer among them, which earned him the nickname of *al-Shaykh al-Akbar*, the Greatest Master. He traveled in Spain, North Africa, Hijaz, Anatolia, Iraq, Palestine, Egypt and Syria.

Ibn al-Fāriḍ, ʿUmar (born in 1181 and died in 1235 in Cairo). Following his father who was an inheritance administrator (*fāriḍ*), he began his career by studying law before turning entirely to sufism. He lived many years as a hermit in the desert and was already venerated as a saint during his lifetime.

Ibn Ḥazm, Abū Muḥammad ʿAlī (born in 994 in Cordoba, died in 1064 in Manta Līshām, an Andalusian village), was a poet, historian, jurist, philosopher, and theologian. He was probably of Christian origin. His father was vizier at the

Spanish Umayyad court and he himself worked for the Umayyads for a while before withdrawing from political life because of the political unrest at that period.

Ibn Khaldūn, Walī al-Dīn ʿAbd al-Raḥmān (born in 1332 in Tunis, died in 1406 in Cairo), was a historian, sociologist, and philosopher. His *Muqaddima* (Prolegomena) is a major contribution to the philosophy of history. He was born in Tunis in an Arab family from Seville, who fled the Reconquista. He received his scholarly education in Tunis. Following the Black Death, which left him without family, he left for Fez, where he was given administrative posts at the Merinid court. He then went to Granada, where he was received at the Nasrid court, then to Bougie, where he became chamberlain while also working as a teacher and preacher. After further stays in Granada and the Maghreb he came to Cairo, the last and most brilliant stage of his career. There he received several appointments as a teacher, head of the *khanqāh* of Baybars, and as a *qadi*. He was sent on a diplomatic mission to Timur during the lathers siege of Damascus.

Ibn Qayyim al-Jawziyya, Shams al-Dīn Abū Bakr Muḥammad (born in 1292 and died in 1350 in Damascus), was a theologian and jurist of the Ḥanbalī school. Together with his Ḥanbalī master Ibn Taymiyya, he spent some time in a Damascus prison. He is the author of many religious and legal studies.

Ibn al-Rūmī, Abū 'l-Ḥasan ʿAlī Ibn al-ʿAbbās (born in 836 and died in 897 in Baghdad), was a poet, also described as a philosopher and a scholar. He was the son of a converted Christian Byzantine father and a Persian mother. He preferred the career of a panegyrist rather than that of a bureaucrat. Because of his *shīʿa* and Muʿtazilit beliefs, he was not always able to enjoy courtly patronage, but had to look for sponsorship among notables elsewhere. Although his poetical production is enormous and varied and not always easy to classify, his work generally belongs to the neo-classicist courtly literary tradition.

Ibn Rushd, Abū 'l-Walīd Muḥammad (born in 1126 in Cordoba, died in 1198 in Marrakesh). Known in the West as Averroës, he was the greatest medieval commentator on Aristotle. Originating from a family of *qadi*s, he too worked as a *qadi* in Seville and in Cordoba. Ibn Ṭufayl introduced him to the Almohad ruler Abū Yaʿqūb Yūsuf in Marrakesh, who eventually sponsored him. Because of pressure from Orthodox scholars, however, Ibn Rushd fell into disgrace for a short period, during which his books were burnt. While he had hardly any Muslim disciples, Ibn Rushd's influence on Western philosophy was particularly strong.

Ibn Sīnā, Abū ʿAlī al-Ḥusayn (born in 980 near Bukhara, died in 1037 in Hamadān/Central Iran). As a physician and a philosopher Ibn Sīnā had a tremendous influence on Islamic as well as on Western culture, where he was named Avicenna. He also had a political career, being for a long period vizier at the Samanid court of Nūḥ Ibn Manṣūr in Bukhara and later in the service of the Buyids in Isfahan and Hamadān.

Ibn Ṭufayl, Abū Bakr Muḥammad (born between 1100 and 1110 in Guadix near Granada, died in 1185/86 in Marrakesh), was a physician and a philosopher. He came from the famous Arab tribe of Qays. In the West he was known as Abubacer. He worked as a physician in Granada, Ceuta, and Tangiers until he was appointed as the court physician of the Almohad ruler Abū Yaʿqūb Yūsuf in Marrakesh. He owes his fame mainly to his philosophical novel, *Ḥayy Ibn Yaqẓān*.

The **Ikhwān al-Ṣafāʾ** were a group of authors who lived in the second half of the 10th century in Basra. They compiled a philosophical encyclopedia consisting of 52 epistles, *Rasāʾil Ikhwān al-Ṣafāʾ*. Although the authors probably belonged to the Shīʿa of Ismāʿīlī orientation, they also had an influence on Sunni scholars.

Imruʾ al-Qays (died around 540) was the most famous Arab pre-Islamic poet. Born as the youngest son of a chieftain of the Kinda tribe, he spent most of his life as a vagrant, hunting, drinking, and composing poetry. After his father's assassination he was introduced by a Ghassanid ruler to the Byzantine emperor Justinian in Constantinople, who is reported to have given him an army in order to help him regain his throne. He died, however, on his way back home, probably poisoned.

al-**Iṣbahānī** (or al-Iṣfahānī), Abū 'l-Faraj (born in 897 in Isfahan, died in 967 in Baghdad) was a historian, a poet, and a littérateur. He was born in Isfahan to a noble Arab family related to the Prophet. He was sponsored by the Hamdanid ruler Sayf al-Dawla in Aleppo and most of all by the Buyids in Baghdad, where he spent most of his life.

al-**Jurjānī**, Abū Bakr ʿAbd al-Qāhir (born in Jurjān along the Caspian Sea, died in 1078 in Jurjān), was known in his lifetime mainly as a grammarian. Posterity, however, remembers him primarily for his theories in literary criticism, which in many respects anticipate modern concepts of art.

al-**Kindī**, Abū Yūsuf Yaʿqūb (born before 800 in Kufa, died in 866 in Baghdad) was called the "Philosopher of the Arabs." He worked at the court of the Abbasid caliphs, to whom he dedicated some of his work. Al-Kindī believed in a harmonization between religion and philosophy.

al-**Maʿarrī**, Abū 'l-ʿAlāʾ Aḥmad (born in 973 and died in 1038 in Maʿarrat al-Nuʿmān in northern Syria), was one of the most outstanding Arab poets. He was born into a family of notables and Shāfiʿī *qadi*s. An early childhood disease left him blind. Little is known about his whereabouts, except for a visit to Baghdad to consult libraries. He spent most of his life in seclusion in his hometown.

al-**Maqrīzī**, Taqīy al-Dīn Abū 'l-ʿAbbās Aḥmad (born in 1364 and died in 1442 in Cairo), originated from a Syrian family of scholars. After a short career in bureaucracy he spent his life as a private scholar and a prolific historian.

al-**Masʿūdī**, Abū 'l-Ḥasan ʿAlī (born in 890 in Baghdad, died in 956 in Fusṭāṭ/Cairo), was a traveler, an encyclopedist, and a historian. He came from an Arab family of noble origin, related to the Prophet. After traveling as far as India, he spent most of his time in Syria and Egypt. His major book *Murūj al-Dhahab* ("Meadows of Gold") is a universal history with a great deal of information about the Abbasid court. He had a great influence on Ibn Khaldūn.

"al-**Mutanabbī**," Abū 'l-Ṭayyib Aḥmad al-Juʿfī (born in 915 in Kufa, died in 954 on his way from Persia to Baghdad), was one of the greatest Arab poets. He took pride in cultivating his Arabic style and therefore spent some time among bedouins. He was the court poet of the Hamdanid ruler Sayf al-Dawla of Aleppo before falling into disgrace because of arrogant behavior. His stay in Egypt at the Ikhshidi court was not successful either. He finally spent some time at the Buyid court in Shiraz and was killed by bedouin robbers on his way back to Baghdad.

al-**Qarṭājannī**, Ḥāzim Abū 'l-Ḥasan (born in 1211 in Cartagena, died in 1285 in Tunis), was a poet, a grammarian, and a literary critic of great originality. After studying in Murcia, Seville, and Granada, he spent some time at the Almohad court in Marrakesh before he was appointed as chancellor at the Hafsid court of Abū Zakariyya in Tunis.

al-**Rāzī**, Abū Bakr Muḥammad (born ca. 854, died in 925 or 935 in Rayy near modern Teheran), was a physician and a philosopher, a common combination at that time. He headed hospitals in Rayy and Baghdad. In the West, where he is known as Rhazes, he is famous for his medical works. His philosophical orientation was Platonic and his ethical ideas were influenced by Socrates.

al-**Shāfiʿī**, Imām Abū ʿAbd Allāh Muḥammad (born in 767 in Palestine or in Yemen, died in 820 in Egypt) originated in a family related to the Prophet. He began his career as a philologist and was also interested in archery. He then studied law in Medina where he attended courses given by Imām Mālik Ibn Ānas, the founder of the Mālikī *madhhab*. He traveled to Yemen, Iraq, and Egypt teaching his doctrine of Islamic law, which eventually became acknowledged as one of the four *madhhab*s of sunnism.

al-**Suhrawardī**, Shihāb al-Dīn Yaḥyā (born in the middle of the 12th century in Suhraward/Persia, died in 1191 in Aleppo), was a famous philosopher and sufi who lived in Isfahan, Baghdad, and Aleppo. There he was sponsored for a while by the ruler al-Malik al-Ẓāhir before he was executed under pressure from the Orthodox ulema.

al-**Tawḥīdī**, ʿAlī Abū Ḥayyān (born between 922 and 932 in Persia or Baghdad, died around 1023 in Shiraz), was a littérateur and a philosopher influenced by Neoplatonism. Perhaps because of his difficult character he could not find princely patronage and had to earn his living as a scribe. At the end of his life he burnt his own books in a fit of bitterness.

Index

Photo Credits

The author wishes to thank Cynthia Robinson for her help with the selection of illustrations, and the following for providing illustrations: Professor Oleg Grabar, photos on pp. 1, 35, 48, 55, 71, 75, 84, 94; Bayerische Staatsbibliothek, Munich, pp. 9 [Cod. arab. 1113 fsr], 18 [Cod. arab. 2569, Bl. 159r]; Professor Tilman Nagel, p. 78.

Archive Doris Behrens-Abouseif: p. 33 (Deutsches Ledermuseum, Offenbach); pp. 45, 49, 54, 105, 125, 142, 150 (photos: B. O'Kane); pp. 58, 153 (Propyläen-Kunstgeschichte [Propyläen-Verlag, Berlin]); p. 59 (Islamic Museum, Cairo [photo: O'Kane]); p. 133 (Louvre, Paris); p. 145 (Staatliche Museen zu Berlin–Preussischer Kulturbesitz, Museum für Islamische Kunst [Photo: G. Niedermeier]); p. 160 (Gayer Anderson Museum, Cairo); p. 179.